The
Diabetes Choice
Cookbook

FOR CANADIANS

Edited by
KATHERINE E. YOUNKER
MBA, RD, Certified Diabetes Educator

Published in cooperation with

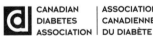

CANADIAN DIABETES ASSOCIATION | ASSOCIATION CANADIENNE DU DIABÈTE

Robert
ROSE

For complete cataloguing information, see page 184.

Disclaimer
The recipes in this book have been carefully tested by our kitchen and our tasters. To the best of our knowledge, they are safe and nutritious for ordinary use and users. For those people with food or other allergies, or who have special food requirements or health issues, please read the suggested contents of each recipe carefully and determine whether or not they may create a problem for you. All recipes are used at the risk of the consumer.

We cannot be responsible for any hazards, loss or damage that may occur as a result of any recipe use.

For those with special needs, allergies, requirements or health problems, in the event of any doubt, please contact your medical adviser prior to the use of any recipe.

Design & Production: PageWave Graphics Inc.
Photography (except for opposite page 161): Mark T. Shapiro

Cover image: Grilled Balsamic Vegetables over Penne (see recipe, page 150)

We acknowledge the financial support of the Government of Canada through the Book Publishing Industry Development Program (BPIDP) for our publishing activities.
Canadä

Published by: Robert Rose Inc.
120 Eglinton Ave. E., Suite 1000, Toronto, Ontario, Canada M4P 1E2
Tel: (416) 322-6552   Fax: (416) 322-6936

Printed in Canada
1 2 3 4 5 6 7 8 9 10   GP   09 08 07 06 05 04 03 02 01

Contents

Foreword

The *Diabetes Choice Cookbook for Canadians* is a collection of recipes from a variety of sources, which together comprise tasty and healthy selections for people affected by diabetes. One of the keys to successfully managing diabetes is meal planning and the majority of people with diabetes and their family members will tell you this is the most challenging task in living day to day with this disease. In fact, most Canadians have eight to nine "standard" meals, which can become uninspiring whether or not they have any health concerns.

Good nutrition and healthy eating receive lots of attention in the press! Canadians with diabetes are aware that what they eat is important not only to help manage blood sugar levels, but also to help prevent complications of diabetes like cardiovascular disease. A balanced intake also plays an important role in the prevention of other diseases like osteoporosis and cancer.

Although not originally designed for those with diabetes, these recipes have been analyzed for nutrient content and on each page you will find the nutrient information (energy in calories, carbohydrate, fiber, protein, fat, saturated fat, cholesterol, and sodium) which will help you to fit these recipes into your meal plan.

Whether you use the *Good Health Eating Guide* system of meal planning, carbohydrate count or attempt to choose a balanced intake, these recipes are for you. The **Canadian Diabetes Association Food Choice Values** are provided for those who follow a meal plan and use the Good Health Eating Guide. **Carbohydrate and fiber** have been included with each recipe to permit easy carbohydrate counting.

You will also find recipe tips, complete meal suggestions and make-ahead information on the recipes contained in this book. Start today and expand your choices in diabetes meal planning. I am sure that you will be able to find a wide range of new family favorites that will make this cookbook one of the staples in managing your meals. Enjoy....

Katherine E. Younker

On Managing Diabetes

Health Canada reports that one in 13 people have diabetes. As of 2001, that means that over 2 million Canadians have diabetes. Diabetes is rapidly becoming the largest public health problem in the Westernized world. As our society becomes more overweight and the population ages, there are many more of us at risk for developing diabetes.

Risk factors for diabetes are many, and if you have been recently diagnosed with diabetes you may have had some of the risk factors identified below:

1. Do I have a family member with diabetes?
There is an increased risk of type 2 diabetes in families with a history of diabetes.

There is a genetic component to type 2 diabetes and this affects your risk of developing the disease. If you have a parent or sibling with type 2 diabetes, your risk is about 40%, but if both of your parents had diabetes, that risk increases to 70%.

2. How old am I?
The risk of developing type 2 diabetes increases with age.

All of our systems age with increasing years. With diabetes, there is a higher rate over age 40 and this increases every decade until the 80s. The longer you live, the greater your chances of developing diabetes.

3. Am I a woman who has delivered a child weighing over 9 lbs (4 kg)?
Having a high birth weight baby may be a risk factor for developing type 2 diabetes later in life.

Women who have given birth to a baby that weighed over 9 lbs at birth may have had gestational diabetes. Gestational diabetes occurs in about 2–4% of all pregnancies, and some people may not have been diagnosed during their pregnancy. Many women with a history of gestational diabetes will develop type 2 diabetes 5–20 years after this pregnancy. In fact, the risk increases with the number of pregnancies, as each additional pregnancy puts more strain on the pancreas.

4. Am I overweight?

About 80% of people with type 2 diabetes are overweight.

Extra body weight makes it harder for your pancreas to function and/or the body becomes more resistant to insulin. Recent studies on prevention of type 2 diabetes found that loss of only 5–10% of body weight can prevent or delay the development of diabetes when coupled with regular physical activity.

What can you do to manage your diabetes and/or help prevent diabetes in family members?

Eating a nutritious low-fat diet, weight maintenance or loss and regular physical activity appear now to be the best methods of preventing diabetes for the population at large. Interestingly, these are the same principles that apply to the prevention of many other chronic diseases as well.

We also know that there are many people who already have elevated blood glucose levels, defined as either **impaired fasting glucose** or **impaired glucose tolerance**. Impaired fasting glucose is defined as a blood glucose (sugar) between 6.1 and 6.9 mmol/L after an overnight fast. Impaired glucose tolerance, defined as blood glucose between 6.1 and 7.0 mmol/L after an overnight fast or values of between 7.8–11.0 two hours after being given a glucose drink containing 75 g of carbohydrate.[1] Studies of people with either of these conditions have found improved eating habits and regular exercise have prevented or delayed the development of diabetes in these individuals.

The diagnosis of diabetes

The diagnosis of diabetes is made when there is a fasting glucose of 7.0 mmol/L or greater on two or more occasions or a glucose level of 11.0 mmol/L or higher, two hours after being given a glucose drink containing 75 g of carbohydrate. People with diabetes may have symptoms such as increased thirst and urination, numbness or tingling in the hands and feet, fatigue, dry mouth and tongue, weight loss or they may exhibit no symptoms at all.

There are three types of diabetes. Type 1 diabetes, found in about 10% of cases, usually occurs in children and young adults and requires insulin for management as the pancreatic cells which produced the insulin are no longer able to produce it. Dietary management and regular activity are additional key treatments.

1. 1998 Clinical Practice Guidelines for the Management of Diabetes in Canada. CMAJ 1998; 159(8 Suppl)

Type 2 diabetes accounts for almost 90% of people diagnosed with diabetes and is usually seen in adults, although there is some recent evidence of its development in children. The pancreas does not produce enough insulin for the individual or the insulin is not used effectively. Type 2 diabetes is managed with a personalized meal plan, physical activity and the addition of oral diabetes medications and/or insulin.

Gestational diabetes occurs in 2–4% of all pregnancies. It is usually managed by diet, exercise and sometimes insulin. Gestational diabetes increases the risk for type 2 diabetes in both the mother and children later in life.

Whatever type of diabetes has been diagnosed, management always includes proper meal planning.

Nutrition Guidelines for Canadians with Diabetes

The Guidelines for the Nutritional Management of Diabetes Mellitus in the New Millennium: A Position Statement, published by the Canadian Diabetes Association provides guiding principles for diabetes meal planning.

The guidelines state the following: "A major goal for diabetes care is to improve glycemic control by balancing food intake with endogenous and/or exogenous insulin levels. For people with type 1 diabetes, insulin doses need to be adjusted to balance with nutritionally adequate food intake and physical activity. For individuals with type 2 diabetes, impaired glucose tolerance or impaired fasting glucose, attention to food portions, and weight management combined with physical activity may help improve glycemic control."[1] The guidelines provide advice on a variety of nutrients of concern to those with diabetes.

CARBOHYDRATE
Recommendations regarding carbohydrate indicate that 50–60% of energy (calories) should be obtained from carbohydrate sources including starch foods, vegetables, fruits, milk products and added

1. The Guidelines for the Nutritional Management of Diabetes Mellitus in the New Millennium: A Position Statement by the Canadian Diabetes Association, Canadian Journal of Diabetes Care, 1999, 23(3) 56–69.

sugar. Added sugars (sucrose, fructose, glucose, etc.) as opposed to those found in vegetables, fruit and milk products may comprise up to 10% of the total daily energy intake.

FIBER
A fiber intake of at least 25–35 g/day is recommended for adults. High fiber food choices are preferred, particularly those with a low glycemic index (such as barley or lentils). Fiber should be chosen from a variety of sources and it is suggested that choosing at least 5–10 g from soluble fiber sources (such as oatmeal or apples) can help to reduce serum (blood) cholesterol.

PROTEIN
Recommendations regarding protein suggest a moderate intake with some emphasis on vegetable protein sources such as beans, lentils and soybeans. An intake of 0.86 g/kg is suggested. For an 80 kg (176 lb) person this would translate into 70 g of protein day, from all sources. A moderate protein intake is helpful in the management of nephropathy (kidney disease) for people with diabetes.

FAT
In keeping with recommendations for all Canadian adults, an intake of less than 30% of energy from fat (ie 600 calories or 65g of fat), and less than 10% from saturated fat (such as processed meats) is recommended. A high fat intake can increase the risk of cardiovascular disease by helping to raise blood lipids (cholesterol), promote weight gain and impair glucose tolerance. Intake of processed foods containing saturated and trans fats should be limited. Monounsaturated fats (from canola, olive and peanut oil) are recommended where possible and polyunsaturated fat should be limited to 10% or less of daily energy. As well, intake of fatty fish containing omega-3 fatty acids (such as salmon and mackerel) at least once a week, has been found to be helpful in lowering triglyceride levels.

ALCOHOL
An alcohol intake of less than 5 % of energy or less than two drinks per day is suggested. This is based on the recommendations for all Canadians. Use of alcohol should be discussed with the diabetes health care team, as it can further aggravate conditions such as hypertension (high blood pressure), dsylipidemia (high blood fat

levels) and liver function. Consumption of alcohol can cause either hyperglycemia (high blood glucose) or hypoglycemia (low blood sugar). Due to the risk of hypoglycemia it is recommended that people with diabetes who take insulin or pills carry with them at all times a readily absorbed source of carbohydrate, inform family and friends regarding the risk and wear identification such as a Medic Alert® bracelet.

SWEETENERS

Sweeteners both "nutritive" (sugar, fructose, aspartame and sugar alcohols such as sorbitol) and "non-nutritive" (acesulfame potassium, sucralose, saccharin and cyclamate) can play a role in the diet of the person with diabetes. Sugar alcohols such as sorbitol, xylitol, mannitol, maltitol, lactitol and isomalt, may be used in moderation with little effect on blood glucose (sugar) levels; in large amounts, they may cause flatulence (gas) and diarrhea. Health Canada has established that aspartame and the "non-nutritive" sweeteners acesulfame potassium, sucralose, saccharin and cyclamate are safe for use and has established an acceptable daily intake. For most individuals with diabetes, moderate use of these sweeteners is acceptable. Use of sweeteners should be discussed with your dietitian on the diabetes health care team.

VITAMINS AND MINERALS

The recommended intake of vitamins and minerals for people with diabetes is the same as for all Canadians. Most individuals can obtain adequate amounts of these nutrients by consuming a well-balanced diet. Some nutrients, such as vitamins C and E, and beta-carotene (which can be converted to vitamin A), may be protective against the development of complications of diabetes. When vitamins and minerals are obtained from plant sources, other components in the plant called "phytochemicals" are consumed as well. These "phytochemicals" are also thought to protect against disease.

Sodium restriction to 2–4 g (2000 to 4000 mg) may help to control hypertension (high blood pressure) in those people who are salt sensitive.

To determine individual requirements, the Canadian Diabetes Association recommends that all persons with diabetes receive nutrition counselling from a registered dietitian. Work with your diabetes health care team to review your dietary intake and a meal plan, which will best suit your lifestyle.

Healthy Eating
and Balanced Blood Glucose (Sugars)

Healthy eating, together with regular activity and if needed, the use of diabetes medication (oral diabetes pills and/or insulin) are the keys to balanced blood glucose (sugars).

The Canadian Diabetes Association recommends several guidelines for meal planning which are important for good health and good glycemic (blood glucose) control. They ask, did you....

- have 3 out of the 4 key food groups at each meal?
  - Starch Foods
  - Fruit & Vegetables
  - Protein Foods
  - Milk

- have 3 meals today, including breakfast?

- have portion sizes that will help you reach or maintain a healthy body weight?

- space your meals 4 to 6 hours apart from each other?

These guidelines can help to start you on the way to healthy eating and balanced blood glucose (sugars).

Although **there are seven Food Choice groups on the Good Health Eating Guide, the four key ones listed above are the most important**. Starch Foods, Fruit & Vegetables and Milk should provide most of the carbohydrate in your diabetes meal plan. Protein Foods are the primary source of protein for most people with diabetes and almost all protein choices contribute some fat to the diet as well. In addition, many foods in the Starch Foods and Milk group can contribute some fat to the diet.

Breakfast is the most important meal of the day, and this is also true for people with diabetes. "Breaking the fast" is essential to provide energy and carbohydrate to begin the day. We need to put some fuel in the tank so that the body can perform during the waking hours. For those with diabetes, not eating breakfast makes it difficult to perform, especially because the only fuel for the brain is glucose. If you have diabetes, which is managed by following a meal plan, skipping breakfast can sometimes make the blood glucose higher. Why? When the body is not supplied with a source of glucose, the brain will signal the body to produce it. The liver then must find sources of glucose, which may include breaking down protein and fat tissue. If your diabetes is managed by oral diabetes medication and/or insulin, skipping breakfast after taking your medication may put you at risk for hypoglycemia or low blood glucose (sugar).

Managing portion sizes is another key to diabetes meal planning. Control or reduction of portion sizes can promote weight loss and glycemic control. Most people with type 2 diabetes are overweight. Recent research has shown that weight control can help to delay type 2 diabetes, which may be an important consideration if other family members do not already have diabetes. Once diabetes is present, loss of body weight in the range of 5–10% has been shown to improve blood glucose (sugar) control and decrease risk factors associated with the complications of diabetes. Reduction and management of fat intake to less than 30% of intake is a successful strategy for long-term weight management.

Managing portion sizes of carbohydrate from meal to meal also contributes directly to the maintenance of euglycemia (normal blood glucose).

Spacing your meals four to six hours apart works to help maintain blood glucose (sugars) and manage appetite. When meals are too close together (less than 4 hours) it may be difficult for most people to achieve a healthy blood glucose before the next meal, as the blood glucose may not have returned to the ideal range (4 to 7 mmol/L). When meals are spaced too far apart (more than 6 hours), the person with diabetes may be at risk for hypoglycemia (low blood sugar) or have difficulty controlling their appetite and thus "forget" to manage portion sizes.

What about snacks? The need for snacks should be reviewed on an individual basis in consultation with the dietitian on your diabetes health care team. For many individuals with diabetes who have a habit of consuming three substantial meals per day, there may not be a need for snacks. Others who work in a physically demanding environment, those who are very active, pregnant or young with a limited stomach capacity, may require between-meal and/or evening snacks to help maintain good blood glucose (sugar) control. The best method of determining this is through home blood glucose (sugar) testing and consultation with your dietitian.

The Little Stuff
vitamins, minerals, fiber and phytochemicals

Vitamins, minerals and fiber are all part of the nutrients we need everyday. When we talk about nutrients such as vitamins and minerals, what do "good" and "excellent" source mean? According to Health Canada each vitamin and mineral has a *Recommended Daily Intake* (RDI) for both children under two and adults. Currently these are based on the 1983 Recommended Nutrient Intakes for Canadians[1], and represents the nutrient intake that meets the needs of most people.

When a recipe indicates it is a good source of a particular nutrient, this means that it contains at least 15% of the RDI, except for vitamin C where it must contain at least 30% of the RDI. An excellent source contains greater than 25% of the RDI for that nutrient or equal to at least 50% in the case of vitamin C. Recipes high in certain nutrients are highlighted in the side bars of particular recipes and many are nutrient packed.

Remember that Vitamins C, E and beta carotene (Vitamin A) are considered to be antioxidant vitamins and may be protective against a number of diseases and potentially some of the complications of diabetes. Choosing foods high in these nutrients is a part of a healthy lifestyle.

Fiber, the indigestible portion of plant foods, is available as both soluble and insoluble. It is an important nutrient for a variety of reasons. Soluble fiber is found in fruits and vegetables, barley, legumes, oats, rye and seeds. When soluble fiber is consumed it slows the digestion of food and may help to control the blood glucose rise after meals. Regular consumption of soluble fiber also helps to lower cholesterol levels. Insoluble fiber, found in cereals, whole grains, beans and lentils, seeds, fruits and vegetables helps to promote regular elimination and may be helpful in reducing cancer risk. Choose high-fiber foods at every meal, where possible. On food labels, high-fiber foods are identified as those that contain 4 g of or more of dietary fiber/serving. Very high fiber foods

---

1. Canadian Food Inspection Agency, Guide to Food Labelling and Advertising, Section VI: Nutrient Content Claims Section 6.4 found at: http://inspection.gc.ca/english/bureau/labeti/guide/6-4e.shtml

contain 6 g or more of dietary fiber/serving and those with 7 g or more can claim to "promote laxation" or "promote regularity". If you need more fiber, choose one of the many high-fiber recipes in this book.

Phytochemicals are substances found in plants which appear to help to increase resistance against disease. A few examples are carotenoids (such as beta carotene in carrots and lycopene in tomatoes), flavonoids (found in berries, celery, onions, grapes, soybeans, whole wheat products), lignans (part of the fiber found in flaxseed), phenolic zacids (found in coffee beans, apples, blueberries, oranges, potatoes and soybeans) and phytoesterols (located in soybeans and lentils).

When choosing to consume food sources of vitamins and minerals rather than supplements, you also obtain the benefit of fiber and phytochemicals. Thus choosing to "eat" your vitamins and minerals offers benefits that no supplement can match.

How to Sweeten?

On average, "added sugars" contain 4 g of carbohydrate per teaspoon, 0 g of protein, 0 g of fat and have an energy value of about 16 calories. (You will find the specific information listed on the nutrition panel on the label of these products.) *The Guidelines for the Nutritional Management of Diabetes Mellitus in the New Millennium*, recommend that added sugars can make up up to 10% of energy intake for a person with diabetes. What does that mean? In practical terms, if you are someone with an energy intake of about 1500 calories per day, about 150 could come from added sugars. This would equal about 9 teaspoons (36 g) of added sugar per day. If your energy intake is about 2000 calories, then 200 calories or about 12 teaspoons (50 g) could come from added sugars.

When choosing to include "added sugars", keep in mind that many packaged products contain added sugar and this should be taken into consideration when choosing how much additional "added sugars" to include. For example, ketchup, salad dressings, creamed corn, coating mixes, cereals and many other items may contain sugar in a variety of forms. Use of products such as these can quickly "use up" those "added sugars".

In preparing recipes, such as the ones contained in these pages, "added sugars" are a part of several recipes in a variety of forms, including granulated white or brown sugar, corn syrup, honey, maple syrup or molasses. When these items are added to a recipe, the carbohydrate content is increased. For example, Pork Stir-Fry with Sweet and Sour Sauce, Snow Peas and Red Peppers (page 113) contains both brown sugar and ketchup, which together contribute about 20 g of carbohydrate or 5 teaspoons of "added sugar" to the recipe. By using a granulated sugar substitute instead of the brown sugar, in this recipe, you can reduce the carbohydrate content by about 15 g (or almost 4 teaspoons) of "added sugar". This may alter the taste slightly, but if you are trying to limit your carbohydrate intake at a meal, it is an easy way to keep within your target.

What should you choose?
That decision depends on several factors:

- Your carbohydrate target for the meal. If you are trying to balance your intake by consuming a certain amount of carbohydrate or food choices from a meal plan, it may be beneficial to use a sugar substitute. If, however, you can adjust your insulin to account for the extra carbohydrate you may choose to leave in the added sugar.

- Personal taste preference. You may wish to choose those products with "added sugars" over those containing "sugar substitutes". If you prefer "added" sugars, you may have to be more particular with your portion sizes to maintain your carbohydrate goals.

- Change of recipe texture or results. In many cases, using a "sugar substitute" in products such as baked goods can alter the recipe texture, color and appearance. When using "sugar substitutes" be sure to follow the manufacturers directions for best results. Most companies have toll free information lines you can call for help.

Fat: Where's it at?

On average, one teaspoon (5 mL) of fat contains 0 g of carbohydrate, 0 g of protein, 5 g of fat and has an energy value of about 45 calories. (You will find the specific information listed on the nutrition panel on the label of these products).The *Guidelines for the Nutritional Management of Diabetes Mellitus in the New Millennium*, recommend that energy from fat contribute no more than 30% of energy intake for a person with diabetes, with less than 10% of energy intake from saturated fat.

In practical terms, if you are someone with an energy intake of about 1500 calories per day, about 450 could come from fat. This would equal about 10 teaspoons (50 mL) of fat (50 g) per day from all sources and of that, 3 teaspoons (15 mL) (or less than 15 grams) from saturated fat. If your energy intake is about 2000 calories, then 600 calories or about 13 teaspoons (65 mL) of fat (65 g) would supply about 30%. Saturated fat should supply less than 4 teaspoons (20 mL) (20 grams) in a 2000 calorie diet.

Remember that fat of various types is found in many foods. Fat is found in protein-containing foods, milk products, dressings and sauces and added to many baked and prepared products. Check the product label to see how much fat is found in the product and choose the lower fat ones.

Most protein-containing foods and milk products contain fat in the form of saturated fat. To limit your intake of saturated fat from these sources, try to:

- Choose lean cuts of meat and trim fat before cooking. Remove poultry skin and avoid food preparation methods such as deep frying, pan frying and those where fat is added.

- Avoid prepared packaged meats, such as deli meats and wieners, unless they are fat reduced.

- Choose low-fat dairy products, like cheeses with a milk fat (M.F.) of 20% or less on the label.

- Choose low-fat milk such as 2%, 1%, or skim milk.

Baked goods, prepared items and fast foods with hydrogenated vegetable oils or shortening contain "trans fatty acids", which are similar to those containing saturated fat and have the same effect on blood lipid (cholesterol) levels. Try to avoid products containing hydrogenated vegetable oils and shortening by:

- Choosing baked goods prepared with soft margarine or vegetable oils such as canola, olive or peanut oil.

- Looking at the labels for products, which contain less than 1 teaspoon (5 g) of fat/serving.

- Preparing your own baked goods at home.

When using fat, try to keep the following in mind:

- Choose oils such as canola, olive or peanut oil.

- Choose soft non-hydrogenated unsaturated margarine in a tub where the polyunsaturated and monounsaturated fats listed on the label are at least 75% of the total fat.

- If you have added fat during cooking, limit the amount of fat you include at the table.

- Nuts and seeds are a good source of unsaturated fat, but are very high in energy. Enjoy them sparingly if you are trying to manage your weight.

- Remember that all fat supplies an equal amount of energy; so even if it is unsaturated, it is wise to limit its use. This is particularly important if you are trying to lose or maintain your weight.

Good Health Eating Guide System

The Good Health Eating Guide (GHEG) System of meal planning is a system known to many individuals with diabetes throughout Canada. First developed in 1982, it replaced the old "Exchange System" formerly used by Canadians with diabetes. Over the last twenty years, it has been updated and revised with the largest change taking place in 1991 when the "Sugars" group was added to the system. Based on Canada's Food Guide and Canada's Guidelines for Healthy Eating, it translates the information into practical meal planning choices for people with diabetes.

Used either as a guide for what to choose at meals or with a calculated meal plan which you have worked out with the dietitian, today the GHEG is still a foundation of diabetes meal planning. In fact, even if you do not have diabetes it is a convenient way of ensuring balanced eating. Many people following weight reduction plans also find it a helpful tool. The Good Health Eating Guide provides information on a variety of foods, by classifying those containing similar macronutrients (carbohydrate, protein, fat and energy [calories]) into one of the seven following Food Choice groups:

■ STARCH FOODS

Starch foods all contribute to a rise in blood glucose and are a key part of a diabetes meal plan. Some choices contain dietary fiber, either as soluble, insoluble, or in combination, which plays an important role in good health and diabetes meal planning.

One choice contains about 15 g carbohydrate, 2 g protein, 0 g fat, and has a 290 kJ (68 calories) energy value.

Examples of one Starch Choice are:

1 slice (1 oz/30 g) bread
½ English muffin
½ hamburger or hot dog bun
1 small plain roll
2 rice cakes
½ medium cob of corn

½ cup (125 mL) cooked cereal
6 soda crackers
1 shredded wheat
½ cup (125 mL) cooked pasta
½ cup (125 mL) cooked barley
½ cup (125 mL) cooked beans
or lentils

🌩 FRUITS & VEGETABLES

All fruits, all juices and some vegetables contain carbohydrate as naturally occurring sugar. They are an important source of vitamins and minerals in the diet and all raise blood sugar levels.

One choice contains about 10 g carbohydrate, 1 g protein, 0 g fat, and has a 190 kJ (44 calories) energy value.

Examples of one Fruit & Vegetables Choice are:

½ medium apple
½ small banana
¼ cantaloupe
10 cherries
½ cup (125 mL) fresh beets
½ cup (125 mL) squash

2 apricots
½ cup (125 mL) blueberries
½ cup (125 mL) cut up fresh fruit
½ grapefruit
½ cup (125 mL) carrots
½ cup (125 mL) mixed vegetables

◆ MILK

All forms of milk contain carbohydrate as lactose, the naturally occurring sugar in milk. Milk is an important source of calcium in the diet of many Canadians and also provides other vitamins and minerals like Vitamin D, phosphorus and riboflavin.

One choice contains about 6 g carbohydrate, 4 g protein, 0 to 4 g fat, and has a 170 kJ (40 calories) to 320 kJ (76 calories) energy value depending upon the type of milk.

Examples of one Milk Choice are:

½ cup (125 mL) milk
¼ cup (50 mL) evaporated milk

½ cup (125 mL) of buttermilk
½ cup (125 mL) plain yogurt

✳ SUGARS

The Sugars group contains foods with added sugar from a variety of sources, which can also be a part of meal planning for diabetes. As with all other foods containing carbohydrate, they contribute to a rise in blood glucose. Nutrition guidelines suggest that **added sugars** can compose up to 10% of the total calories in the diet of people with diabetes. Added sugars contribute little in the way of nutrients to meal planning, but when substituted for other carbohydrates increase meal plan flexibility and choice.

One choice contains about 10 g of carbohydrate, 0 g of protein, and 0 g of fat and has 168 kJ (40 calories) energy value.

Examples of one Sugars choice are:

2 tsp (10 mL) white
or brown sugar

2 small sweet pickles (gherkins)

2 hard candies

½ popsicle

⅓ cup (75 mL) regular
cranberry cocktail

1 large bubble gum

1 tbsp (15 mL) regular jam, jelly
or marmalade

2 tbsp (25 mL) sweet relish

4 jelly beans

2 marshmallows

2 tsp (10 mL) honey, molasses,
maple or corn syrup

½ cup (125 mL) regular soft drink

⊘ PROTEIN FOODS

Protein Foods are made up of choices like fish, lean meat, poultry, cheese and those from plant sources such as peanut butter, soybeans, tofu and lentils. Protein foods, except for lentils and other legumes, contain no carbohydrate and do not directly affect blood glucose levels. In addition to providing protein, many meats provide iron and some types of fish provide fats such as omega-3 fatty acids. Vegetable proteins may contain plant sterols and phytochemicals.

One choice contains about 0 g carbohydrate, 7 g protein, 3 g fat, and has a 230 kJ (55 calories) energy value.

Examples of one Protein choice are:

1 oz (30 g) fish

3 medium clams, mussels, scallops

½ block (70 g) tofu

1 slice low-fat (7% m.f.) cheese

1 slice (1 oz/30 g) heart or liver

1 slice (1 oz/30 g) lean meat
or chicken

¼ cup (50 mL) canned salmon

5 large shrimp

1 medium egg

¼ cup (50 mL) 2% cottage cheese

½ chop (1½ oz/40 g), with bone

2 tbsp (25 mL) lean ground
chicken or beef

▲ FATS & OILS

Fats & Oils add energy to the diet and some provide a source of essential fatty acids. While fats contribute energy to the diet, it is very important for people with diabetes to watch both the amount of fat and type of fat they choose. Monounsaturated fats found in some plant oils (canola, olive and peanut) are the preferred choice and both saturated and polyunsaturated fats should be limited to about 10% of energy intake or the equivalent of about 4 to 5 Fats & Oils choices (or teaspoons) per day. Soft, non-hydrogenated margarines are a better choice as a spread and in cooking.

One choice contains about 0 g protein, 5 g fat, 0 g carbohydrate and has a 190 kJ (45 calories) energy value.

Examples of one Fats & Oils choice are:

1 tsp (5 mL) oil

2 tbsp (25 mL) low-calorie salad dressing

1 tsp (5 mL) margarine

1 tbsp (15 mL) cheese spread*

1 slice bacon, side, crisp*

1 tbsp (15 mL) dried unsweetened coconut*

10 peanuts

1 tbsp (15 mL) sunflower seeds (shelled)

5 tsp (25 mL) pine nuts

7 black olives

1 tbsp (15 mL) whipping cream*

2 tbsp (25 mL) sour cream (12% m.f.)*

These items are sources of saturated fat.

⊡⊡ EXTRAS

The Extras add variety to diabetes meal planning. The foods in this group include vegetables and other items, which are both low in calories and carbohydrate. The Extra vegetables in this section can provide valuable vitamins, minerals and phytochemicals in the meal plan of someone with diabetes. As most of these vegetables are low in carbohydrate, when eaten in small quantities (less than ½ cup or 125 mL), they do not have to be counted in your meal plan.

One choice usually contains less than 2.5 g carbohydrate, 0 g protein, 0 g fat, and has a 60 kJ (15 calories) energy.

Examples of one Extras choice are shown below:

Extra Vegetables

Artichokes

Broccoli

Cauliflower

Lettuce

Peppers, green, red and yellow

Asparagus

Cabbage

Cucumber

Mushrooms

Spinach

Extras

Garlic

Mineral water

Sugar-free soft drinks

Vinegar

Coffee Flavorings and Extracts

Lemon juice

Sugar-free gelatin desserts

Tea

Spices

The Good Health Eating Guide system is composed of both a poster and resource book. These are available from:

• Your health care team at your local diabetes education center;

• A dietitian at your local hospital or community health center;

• The provincial branch or national office of the Canadian Diabetes Association.

Carbohydrate Counting

Carbohydrate counting is a method of meal management used by people with diabetes as an alternative to following a meal plan. People choosing to carbohydrate count are often those people who use a rapid acting insulin, which they can adjust depending on their carbohydrate consumption. This increases meal flexibility and usually allows the person with diabetes to "eat to appetite", as many of us have day-to-day fluctuations in our intake based on a variety of factors.

One advantage of the newer rapid acting insulins is that they can be taken after meals, which permits people to judge how much insulin to take based on how much they have actually eaten.

Is there a downside to carbohydrate counting?

Sometimes people who choose to carbohydrate count "forget" about good nutrition. This can occur when they view their increased meal flexibility as an opportunity to make food choices that they may have viewed with caution before.

For example, choosing to eat high-fat, high-carbohydrate desserts regularly may mean not making more nutritious choices such as fresh fruit with meals. What are the consequences of this? A large amount of short-acting insulin may be required to return the blood glucose to a "normal" level and over time this may lead to weight gain. Making these choices can also impact on weight and blood fat (cholesterol) levels. Lastly, substituting low-nutrient foods for healthier selections may deprive the body of a number of essential nutrients such as calcium, vitamins A and C, fiber and a whole host of others.

WORKING WITH A DIETITIAN

If you are thinking about using carbohydrate counting as a method of meal planning, it is a good idea to see the dietitian from your diabetes health care team for help in getting started. Together you can review the essentials of carbohydrate counting, look at your regular intake to determine an appropriate carbohydrate/insulin ratio and work through any pitfalls which result when you begin.

What are the principles of carbohydrate counting?

Carbohydrate found in foods is known to be the primary source of glucose in the blood. Although both of the other "macronutrients", protein and fat, can be turned into glucose, this will not usually occur, except when there is inadequate carbohydrate available to the body for energy.

There are several forms of carbohydrate, some which contribute to blood glucose and some which do not. These are sugars, starch, dietary fiber and "sugar alcohols". The latter are usually seen in products developed for people with diabetes such as "no sugar added" candies and small amounts sometimes occur naturally in foods.

Dietary fiber, primarily undigested by the body, is one of the components of carbohydrate which does not raise the blood glucose. Therefore when counting carbohydrate, it is important to remove the dietary fiber from the total carbohydrate to determine the *available carbohydrate. Available carbohydrate is the carbohydrate which will contribute to a rise in blood glucose.*

If you plan your meals and snacks by counting carbohydrate, there are two ways to do this:

METHOD I

Use the Canadian Diabetes Association Food Choice Values and Symbols system. With this method, all the nutrient information affecting the available carbohydrate has been considered before determining the Food Choice Values and Symbols.

Carbohydrate is found in four of the seven food choice groups on the Good Health Eating Guide. Here is the amount of carbohydrate in 1 Food Choice in each of the seven Food Choice groups.

Food Choices	Grams of Carbohydrate
1 ■ Starch	15
1 ● Fruits & Vegetables	10
1 ◆ Milk	6
1 ✳ Sugars	10
1 ● Protein	0
1 ▲ Fats & Oils	0
1 ❖ Extras	0

If you are using a recipe such as Spicy Rice, Bean and Lentil Casserole (page 138) where the Food Choice Value listed is 3 ■ + 1 ● + 1½ ●, you can determine the available carbohydrate by doing the following: look at the Food Choices for each and multiply the grams (g) of carbohydrate per food group, then add them together to obtain a total.

Food Choice	Grams of carbohydrate per choice grams (g)	Available carbohydrate
3 ■ x	15	= 45 g
1 ● x	10	= 10 g
1½ ● x	0	= 0 g
Available carbohydrate		= 55 g

METHOD 2

You may also count carbohydrate by looking at the nutrient information listed on for the recipes. Using this method, take the amount of carbohydrate listed and subtract the fiber. This provides you with the amount of "available" carbohydrate per recipe.

For example, the nutrition information for the Spicy Rice, Bean and Lentil Casserole recipe (page 138) indicates:

Energy	341 kcal
Carbohydrates	65 g
Fiber	11 g
Protein	17 g
Fat, total	3 g
Fat, saturated	0 g
Sodium	362 mg
Cholesterol	0 mg
Carbohydrate	65 g
Fiber	11 g
Available carbohydrate	54 g

There is a slight difference between both methods due to rounding of the nutrients to whole numbers. The differences are generally small and do not make one method better than the other, but choice may be based on personal preference and comfort.

Using this information together with the carbohydrate from the other foods in your meal you can estimate the total amount of **available carbohydrate** and determine how much insulin to take based on your **carbohydrate to insulin** ratio. Once again, it is important to work with the dietitian on your diabetes health care team to determine your individual carbohydrate to insulin ratio and to become comfortable with this method of meal planning.

Remember when using this method, don't forget about healthy eating and good nutrition.

Glycemic Index

The "glycemic index" is a measure of the body's response to consuming different types of carbohydrate foods. After eating carbohydrate containing foods, blood glucose levels rise and the extent of that rise is called the "glycemic response". The "glycemic index" is a way to categorize the glycemic response of a certain food in comparison to a standard, usually glucose or white bread. The effect of each of these foods on blood glucose has been given a value. (See table below.)

There are many factors which contribute to a food's glycemic effect and this may be due in part to the soluble fiber and chemical compositon of the food, how slowly or quickly the food is digested, how the food has been prepared and whether the food is eaten alone or as part of a meal.

For people with diabetes, this means that by choosing foods that have a low glycemic index more often, there may be less of a rise in blood glucose after meals or snacks. In some instances, where people have regularly chosen low glycemic index foods, they have required less insulin. There is also some research indicating that choosing foods which have a low glycemic index may decrease the risk of developing type 2 diabetes.

GLYCEMIC INDEX OF SELECTED FOODS
Lowest Glycemic Index to High Glycemic Index

Food	GI	Food	GI
Pearl barley	25	Boxed macaroni and cheese	64
Legumes	25–48	Rye crisp bread	65
Tomato soup	38	Couscous	65
Spaghetti	41	Shredded wheat	69
Parboiled rice	47	Whole wheat bread	69
Bran Buds with Psyllium®	47	White wheat bread	70
Bulgur (cracked wheat)	48	Cornmeal	70
Red River Cereal®	49	Mashed potato	70–83
Chocolate	49	Corn chips	73
Rye kernel-pumpernickel bread	50	Puffed Wheat®	74
Yams	51	French fries	75
Oat Bran	55	Jelly beans	80
Polished rice	56	Cornflakes®	84
Pita Bread	57	Puffed Rice®	86
Oatmeal	61	Rice cakes	88
White/whole/canned potatoes	61	Glucose	100

References: Wolever, T.M.S. , Glycemic Index Workshop, 2000.

Recipe Analysis

The recipes were analyzed using the Nutriwatch Nutrient Analysis Program (Canadian Nutrient file 1997), Version 6.120E, Delphi 1, copyright 2000, Elizabeth Warwick. Where necessary additional data was supplemented using the USDA database on line.

Analysis information was based on:

Imperial measures and weights were used, except where metric measurements were listed.

The larger number of servings were used when there was a range.

The first ingredient and amount were used where alternatives were specified.

Optional ingredients were not included.

Calculations including meat and poultry used lean portions without skin.

As indicated, 2% milk and regular cheese have been used in the majority of these recipes, except where specified otherwise. In most instances, you should be able to successfully use lower-fat milk and low-fat cheese to further reduce the fat content.

Nutrient values were rounded to the nearest whole number for presentation in the text. In calculation of the Canadian Diabetes Association Food Choice Values the actual nutrient values were used, prior to rounding.

Soft margarine and canola oil were used in recipe analysis where the type of fat was not specified.

EDITOR'S NOTE: No sugar added yogurt is listed in the side bars to complete a number of meals. Your personal carbohydrate goals for a meal may permit you to include a regular fruit flavored yogurt instead.

Appetizers

Appetizers are a delicious way to begin a meal or entertain guests. Many can be prepared ahead and "cooked" just when guest arrive, allowing the host or hostess to enjoy company rather than "fuss" with food.

A collection of appetizers together with low-fat crackers or whole grain bread can actually be used in combination to make a meal.

When preparing to entertain keep in mind, some friends with diabetes may need to watch the timing of meals and snacks.

It is always prudent for hosts to provide both alcoholic and non-alcoholic drinks to provide choice for those who need to drive or some who may have to limit alcohol for medical reasons. Sugar-free soft drinks combined with Crystal-Light® or light (reduced carbohydrate) cranberry cocktail are delicious alcohol-free alternatives.

❖

Buy snow peas that are
firm and crisp, and have
no blemishes.

◆

Medium-sized scallops
would also be delicious
for this very sophisticated
hors d'oeuvre.

Shrimp and Snow Pea Tidbits

16	snow peas	16
2 tsp	vegetable oil	10 mL
1 tsp	crushed garlic	5 mL
1 tbsp	chopped fresh parsley	15 mL
16	medium shrimp, peeled, deveined, tail left on	16

1. Steam or microwave snow peas until barely
tendercrisp. Rinse with cold water. Drain and
set aside.

2. In nonstick skillet, heat oil; sauté garlic,
parsley and shrimp just until shrimp turn pink,
3 to 5 minutes.

3. Wrap each snow pea around shrimp; fasten
with toothpick. Serve warm or cold.

MAKE AHEAD ◆ If serving cold, prepare and
refrigerate early in day.

PER SERVING

½ ⊘ Protein Choice

1 ◆◆ Extra Choice

Calories 39
Carbohydrates . . . . . 1 g
Fiber . . . . 0 g
Protein . . . . 4 g
Fat, total . . . . 2 g
Fat, saturated . . . . 0 g
Sodium . . . . 27 mg
Cholesterol . . . . . 28 mg

Serves 4 to 6 or
makes 18 hors
d'oeuvres

Preheat broiler

Baking sheet sprayed
with nonstick
vegetable spray

TIP

Tender beef is delicious
with this sweet
oriental sauce.

Oriental Chicken Wrapped Mushrooms

1 tbsp	rice wine vinegar	15 mL
1 tbsp	vegetable oil	15 mL
2 tbsp	soya sauce	25 mL
1 tsp	crushed garlic	5 mL
2 tbsp	finely chopped onion	25 mL
1 tsp	sesame oil	5 mL
2 tbsp	water	25 mL
2 tbsp	brown sugar	25 mL
½ tsp	sesame seeds (optional)	2 mL
¾ lb	boneless skinless chicken breast	375 g
18	medium mushroom caps (without stems)	18

1. In bowl, combine vinegar, oil, soya sauce, garlic, onion, sesame oil, water, sugar, and sesame seeds (if using); mix well.

2. Cut chicken into strips about 3 inches (8 cm) long and 1 inch (2.5 cm) wide to make 18 strips. Add to bowl and marinate for 20 minutes, stirring occasionally.

3. Wrap each chicken strip around mushroom; secure with toothpick. Place on baking sheet. Broil for approximately 5 minutes or until chicken is no longer pink inside. Serve immediately.

MAKE AHEAD ◆ Refrigerate chicken in marinade early in day. Wrap chicken around mushroom caps and broil just before serving.

PER SERVING

½	✳	Sugar Choice
2	◉	Protein Choices
1	✦✦	Extra Choice

Calories 130
Carbohydrates . . . . . 7 g
Fiber . . . . 0 g
Protein . . . . 15 g
Fat, total . . . . 5 g
Fat, saturated . . . . 1 g
Sodium . . . . 329 mg
Cholesterol . . . . . 36 mg

Preheat oven to
400°F (200°C)

This filling can be used
to stuff medium
mushrooms. Just remove
the mushroom stems.

◆

You can reduce the
fat content of this recipe
by choosing low-fat
cheeses. One-eighth of
the recipe (or 4 cherry
tomatoes) is a good
source of vitamin C.

Warm Cherry Tomatoes Stuffed with Garlic and Cheese

24	cherry tomatoes	24
½ cup	dry bread crumbs	125 mL
2 tbsp	chopped green onion	25 mL
½ tsp	chopped garlic	2 mL
2 tbsp	chopped fresh parsley	25 mL
1 tbsp	margarine, melted	15 mL
⅓ cup	shredded mozzarella cheese	75 mL
1 tbsp	grated Parmesan cheese	15 mL

1. Cut slice from top of each tomato; carefully scoop out seeds and most of the pulp.

2. In bowl, combine bread crumbs, onion, garlic, parsley, margarine and mozzarella until well mixed.

3. Spoon into tomatoes; sprinkle with Parmesan. Place on baking sheet and bake for approximately 10 minutes or until stuffing is golden.

MAKE AHEAD ◆ Make early in day and refrigerate. Bake just before serving.

PER SERVING

½   ◪   Fruit & Vegetable Choice

½   ◪   Protein Choice

½   ▲   Fat & Oil Choice

1   ✚   Extra Choice

Calories 87
Carbohydrates . . . . . 8 g
Fiber . . . . 1 g
Protein . . . . 4 g
Fat, total . . . . 5 g
Fat, saturated . . . . 2 g
Sodium . . . . 134 mg
Cholesterol . . . . . 10 mg

Goat cheese, also known
as chèvre, comes in a
variety of shapes ranging
from logs to pyramids
and discs. Some are
sprinkled with herbs and
spices throughout.
Use any variety.

◆

Serve also as a dip
or serve on celery
sticks or in hollow
cherry tomatoes.

Smoked Salmon and Goat Cheese Cucumber Slices

3 oz	smoked salmon, diced	75 g
3 oz	goat cheese	75 g
2 tbsp	2% yogurt	25 mL
½ tsp	lemon juice	2 mL
4 tsp	chopped fresh dill (or ½ tsp [2 mL] dried dillweed)	20 mL
25	slices (¼-inch [5 mm] thick) cucumber	25

1. Reserve about 25 bits of salmon for garnish.

2. In bowl or using food processor, combine goat cheese, yogurt, remaining salmon, lemon juice and dill; mix with fork or using on/off motion just until combined but not puréed.

3. Place spoonful of filling on each cucumber slice. Garnish with bit of reserved salmon.

MAKE AHEAD ◆ Prepare and refrigerate mixture up to a day before. Place on cucumber slices just before serving.

PER SERVING

1	⊘ Protein Choice
½	▲ Fat & Oil Choice
1	✚ Extra Choice

Calories	92
Carbohydrates	2 g
Fiber	0 g
Protein	8 g
Fat, total	6 g
Fat, saturated	4 g
Sodium	156 mg
Cholesterol	19 mg

Preheat oven to
425°F (220°C)

Baking sheet sprayed
with vegetable spray

TIP

If using fresh spinach, use
half the package (5 oz
[125 g]), wash and cook
with water clinging to
leaves until wilted and
cooked (approximately
3 minutes). Drain, rinse
with cold water, squeeze
out excess moisture and
chop. Goat cheese can
replace the feta cheese.

Greek Egg Rolls
with Spinach and Feta

2 tsp	vegetable oil	10 mL
2 tsp	minced garlic	10 mL
¾ cup	diced onions	175 mL
1⅔ cup	diced mushrooms	400 mL
1 tsp	dried oregano	5 mL
Half	package (10 oz [300 g]) frozen chopped spinach, thawed and drained	Half
2 oz	feta cheese, crumbled	50 g
10	egg roll wrappers	10

1. In nonstick skillet, heat oil over medium-high heat. Add garlic, onions, mushrooms and oregano; cook for 5 minutes or until softened. Add spinach and feta; cook, stirring, for 2 minutes or until well mixed and cheese melts.

2. Keeping rest of egg roll wrappers covered with a cloth to prevent drying out, put one wrapper on work surface with a corner pointing towards you. Put 2 tbsp (25 mL) of the filling in the center. Fold the lower corner up over the filling, fold the two side corners in over the filling and roll the bundle away from you. Place on prepared pan and repeat until all wrappers are filled. Bake for 12 to 14 minutes until browned, turning the egg rolls at the halfway point.

MAKE AHEAD ◆ Prepare early in the day, cover and keep refrigerated until ready to bake.

PER SERVING

1	■ Starch Choice
½	◧ Fruit & Vegetable Choice
½	◎ Protein Choice

Calories 132
Carbohydrates . . . . 22 g
Fiber . . . . 1 g
Protein . . . . 5 g
Fat, total . . . . 3 g
Fat, saturated . . . . 1 g
Sodium . . . . 251 mg
Cholesterol . . . . . . 8 mg

Asparagus and Leek Soup (page 47) ➤

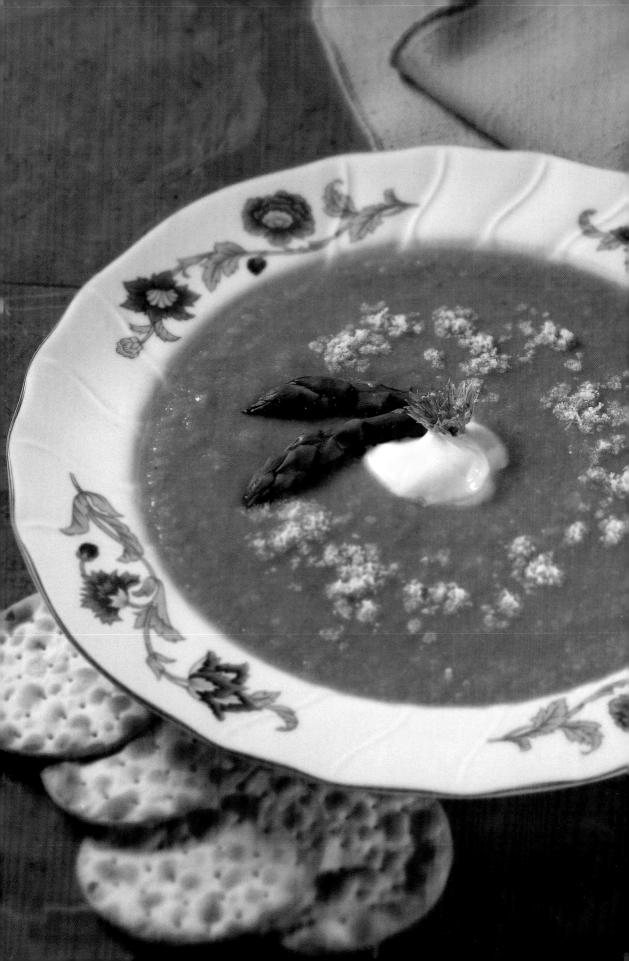

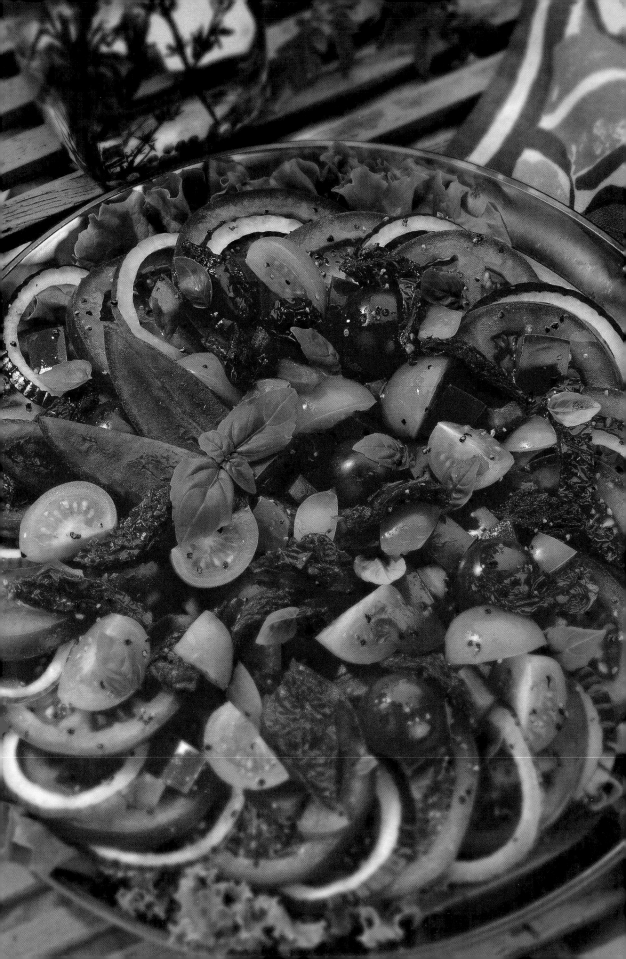

If suggested seafood is not used, try a firm white fish such as swordfish, haddock, or monkfish.

◆

A combination of seafood together with these vegetables make this appetizer packed with nutrients. It is an excellent source of vitamins C and B$_{12}$ and a good source of vitamin A, magnesium, phosphorus, iron and niacin.

Seafood Garlic Antipasto

1 lb	scallops, squid or shrimp, or a combination, cut into pieces	500 g
¾ cup	chopped snow peas	175 mL
¾ cup	chopped red peppers	175 mL
½ cup	diced tomatoes	125 mL
⅓ cup	chopped red onions	75 mL
⅓ cup	minced coriander or dill	75 mL
¼ cup	sliced black olives	50 mL
3 tbsp	lemon juice	45 mL
2 tbsp	olive oil	25 mL
1 ½ tsp	minced garlic	7 mL
	Pepper to taste	

1. In a nonstick skillet sprayed with vegetable spray, cook the seafood over medium-high heat for 3 minutes, or until just done. Drain excess liquid, if any, and place seafood in serving bowl. Let cool slightly.

2. Add snow peas, red peppers, tomatoes, red onions, coriander and olives; mix well. Whisk together lemon juice, olive oil, garlic; pour over seafood mixture. Add pepper to taste. Chill for 1 hour before serving.

MAKE AHEAD ◆ Prepare early in the day and keep refrigerated. Mix before serving.

PER SERVING

½ 🥬 Fruit & Vegetable Choice

2½ 🥬 Protein Choices

Calories	150
Carbohydrates	7 g
Fiber	1 g
Protein	17 g
Fat, total	6 g
Fat, saturated	1 g
Sodium	137 mg
Cholesterol	115 mg

◄ Four-Tomato Salad (page 59)

Tuna packed in water
is a great substitute
for salmon.

♦

You can also use the
mixture as a dip if you
purée it until smooth.

♦

Serve 2 whole halves
as a light lunch.

Salmon Swiss Cheese English Muffins

1	can (7½ oz [220 g]) salmon, drained	1
¼ cup	light mayonnaise	50 mL
2 tbsp	chopped green onion	25 mL
2 tbsp	chopped red onion	25 mL
2 tbsp	diced celery	25 mL
2 tbsp	chopped fresh dill (or 1 tsp [5 mL] dried dillweed)	25 mL
2 tsp	lemon juice	10 mL
4	English muffins, split in half and toasted	4
⅓ cup	shredded Swiss cheese	75 mL

1. In food processor, combine salmon, mayonnaise, green and red onions, celery, dill and lemon juice. Using on/off motion, process just until chunky but not puréed.

2. Divide salmon mixture over muffins and spread evenly. Sprinkle with cheese. Broil just until cheese melts, approximately 2 minutes. To serve, slice each muffin into quarters.

MAKE AHEAD ♦ Make and refrigerate salmon mixture up to a day before. Stir before spreading on muffins.

PER SERVING

1	■	Starch Choice
1	◿	Protein Choice
½	▲	Fat & Oil Choice

Calories 149
Carbohydrates . . . . 15 g
Fiber . . . . 0 g
Protein . . . . 8 g
Fat, total . . . . 7 g
Fat, saturated . . . . 2 g
Sodium . . . . 213 mg
Cholesterol . . . . . 14 mg

Adjust the chili powder
to your taste.

◆

Serve with pita bread,
vegetables or crackers.

Avocado, Tomato and Chili Guacamole

Half	avocado, peeled	Half
¾ tsp	crushed garlic	4 mL
2 tbsp	chopped green onions	25 mL
I tbsp	lemon juice	15 mL
¼ cup	finely diced sweet red pepper	50 mL
½ cup	chopped tomato	125 mL
Pinch	chili powder	Pinch

I. In bowl, combine avocado, garlic, onions, lemon juice, red pepper, tomato and chili powder; mash with fork, mixing well.

MAKE AHEAD ◆ Make early in day and squeeze more lemon juice over top to prevent discoloration. Refrigerate. Stir just before serving.

PER SERVING

½ ◢ Fruit & Vegetable Choice

I ✦✦ Extra Choice

Calories	35
Carbohydrates	3 g
Fiber	I g
Protein	I g
Fat, total	3 g
Fat, saturated	0 g
Sodium	5 mg
Cholesterol	0 mg

Serves 6 to 8

Preheat oven to 350°F
(180°C)

Small casserole dish

The three cheeses in this
recipe make it a good
source of calcium.
Served with French
bread, this recipe can
make a delicious lunch.
To complete the meal
choose ✦✦ Extra
Vegetables and ◢ Fruit
& Vegetable choices
such as a fresh pear.

◆

Serve over French bread
or with vegetables.

Hot Three-Cheese Dill Artichoke Bake

1	can (14 oz [398 mL]) artichoke hearts, drained and halved	1
½ cup	shredded part-skim mozzarella cheese (about 2 oz [50 g])	125 mL
⅓ cup	shredded Swiss cheese (about 1 ½ oz [35 g])	75 mL
⅓ cup	minced fresh dill (or 1 tsp [5 mL] dried)	75 mL
¼ cup	light sour cream	50 mL
3 tbsp	light mayonnaise	45 mL
1 tbsp	freshly squeezed lemon juice	15 mL
1 tsp	minced garlic	5 mL
Pinch	cayenne pepper	Pinch
1 tbsp	grated Parmesan cheese	15 mL

1. In a food processor, combine artichoke hearts, mozzarella and Swiss cheeses, dill, sour cream, mayonnaise, lemon juice, garlic and cayenne. Process on and off just until combined but still chunky. Place in a small casserole dish. Sprinkle with Parmesan cheese.

2. Bake uncovered 10 minutes. Broil 3 to 5 minutes just until top is slightly browned. Serve warm with crackers.

MAKE AHEAD ◆ Prepare up to 1 day in advance. Bake just before serving.

PER SERVING

1	◢ Protein Choice
1	▲ Fat & Oil Choice
1	✦✦ Extra Choice

Calories 116
Carbohydrates . . . . . 3 g
Fiber . . . . 0 g
Protein . . . . 8 g
Fat, total . . . . 8 g
Fat, saturated . . . . 4 g
Sodium . . . . 218 mg
Cholesterol . . . . . 21 mg

Creamy Sun-Dried Tomato Dip

4 oz	dry-packed sun-dried tomatoes	125 g
¾ cup	5% ricotta cheese	175 mL
½ cup	chopped fresh parsley	125 mL
⅓ cup	basic vegetable stock (see recipe, page 46) or water	75 mL
3 tbsp	chopped black olives	45 mL
2 tbsp	olive oil	25 mL
2 tbsp	toasted pine nuts	25 mL
2 tbsp	grated Parmesan cheese	25 mL
1 tsp	minced garlic	5 mL

1. In a small bowl, pour boiling water to cover over sun-dried tomatoes. Let stand 15 minutes. Drain and chop.

2. In a food processor combine sun-dried tomatoes, ricotta, parsley, stock, olives, olive oil, pine nuts, Parmesan and garlic; process until well combined but still chunky. Makes 1¾ cups (425 mL).

MAKE AHEAD ◆ Prepare up to 3 days in advance.

PER SERVING

1	Fruit & Vegetable Choice
½	Protein Choice
1	Fat & Oil Choice

Calories	 111
Carbohydrates	.... 10 g
Fiber	.... 0 g
Protein	.... 6 g
Fat, total	.... 6 g
Fat, saturated	.... 2 g
Sodium	.... 356 mg
Cholesterol	...... 8 mg

Creamy Pesto Dip

TIPS

To toast pine nuts, put in nonstick skillet over medium-high heat for 3 minutes, stirring occasionally. Or put them on a baking sheet and toast in a 400°F (200°C) oven for 5 minutes. Whichever method you choose, watch carefully — nuts burn quickly.

◆

If basil is not available, use parsley or spinach leaves.

◆

When choosing ■ Starch Choices to serve with this dip, look for crisps or crackers with less than 2 g of fat/serving.

I cup	well-packed basil leaves	250 mL
2 tbsp	toasted pine nuts	25 mL
2 tbsp	grated Parmesan cheese	25 mL
2 tbsp	olive oil	25 mL
2 tsp	lemon juice	10 mL
I tsp	minced garlic	5 mL
½ cup	5% ricotta cheese	125 mL
¼ cup	light sour cream	50 mL

I. Put basil, pine nuts, Parmesan, olive oil, lemon juice and garlic in food processor; process until finely chopped, scraping sides of bowl down once. Add ricotta and sour cream and process until smooth. Serve with pita or tortilla crisps, or fresh vegetables.

MAKE AHEAD ◆ Prepare early in the day and keep covered and refrigerated.

PER SERVING

½ ◉ Protein Choice

I   ▲ Fat & Oil Choice

Calories 72
Carbohydrates . . . . . 2 g
Fiber . . . . 0 g
Protein . . . . 3 g
Fat, total . . . . 6 g
Fat, saturated . . . . 2 g
Sodium . . . . 53 mg
Cholesterol . . . . . . 9 mg

Serves 8 to 10

9- by 5-inch (2 L) loaf pan lined with plastic wrap

PER SERVING

½ 🍃 Fruit & Vegetable Choice

½ 🖉 Protein Choice

½ 🔺 Fat & Oil Choice

Calories 80
Carbohydrates . . . . . 6 g
Fiber . . . . 1 g
Protein . . . . 4 g
Fat, total . . . . 5 g
Fat, saturated . . . . 2 g
Sodium . . . . 124 mg
Cholesterol . . . . . 13 mg

Leek Mushroom Cheese Pâté

2 tsp	vegetable oil	10 mL
1½ tsp	minced garlic	7 mL
1½ cups	chopped leeks	375 mL
½ cup	finely chopped carrots	125 mL
12 oz	oyster or regular mushrooms, thinly sliced	375 g
2 tbsp	sherry or white wine	25 mL
2 tbsp	chopped fresh dill (or 2 tsp [10 mL] dried)	25 mL
1½ tsp	dried oregano	7 mL
¼ tsp	coarsely ground black pepper	1 mL
2 oz	feta cheese, crumbled	50 g
2 oz	light cream cheese	50 g
½ cup	5% ricotta cheese	125 mL
2 tsp	freshly squeezed lemon juice	10 mL
2 tbsp	chopped fresh dill	25 mL

1. In a large nonstick frying pan sprayed with vegetable spray, heat oil over medium-high heat. Add garlic, leeks and carrots; cook 3 minutes, stirring occasionally. Stir in mushrooms, sherry, dill, oregano and pepper; cook, stirring occasionally, 8 to 10 minutes or until carrots are tender and liquid is absorbed. Remove from heat.

2. Transfer vegetable mixture to a food processor. Add feta, cream cheese, ricotta and lemon juice; purée until smooth. Spoon into prepared loaf pan. Cover and chill until firm.

3. Invert onto serving platter; sprinkle with chopped dill. Serve with crackers, bread or vegetables.

MAKE AHEAD ◆ Prepare up to 2 days in advance.

White navy pea beans can also be used. If you cook your own dry beans, ½ cup (125 mL) dry yields approximately 1½ cups (375 mL) of cooked beans.

◆

The red pepper in this recipe makes it a good source of vitamin C.

Tuna and White Bean Spread

1 cup	canned, cooked white kidney beans, drained	250 mL
1	can (6.5 oz [184 g]) tuna in water, drained	1
1½ tsp	minced garlic	7 mL
2 tbsp	lemon juice	25 mL
2 tbsp	light mayonnaise	25 mL
¼ cup	5% ricotta cheese	50 mL
3 tbsp	minced red onions	45 mL
¼ cup	minced fresh dill (or 1 tsp [5 mL] dried)	50 mL
1 tbsp	grated Parmesan cheese	15 mL
¼ cup	diced red pepper	50 mL

1. Place beans, tuna, garlic, lemon juice, mayonnaise and ricotta in food processor; pulse on and off until combined but still chunky. Place in serving bowl.

2. Stir onions, dill, Parmesan and red pepper into bean mixture.

MAKE AHEAD ◆ Prepare up to a day ahead; keep covered and refrigerated. Stir before using.

PER SERVING

½	■ Starch Choice
1	◨ Protein Choice

Calories 88
Carbohydrates . . . . . 9 g
Fiber . . . . 0 g
Protein . . . . 7 g
Fat, total . . . . 3 g
Fat, saturated . . . . 1 g
Sodium . . . . 52 mg
Cholesterol . . . . . 10 mg

Soups

Soups come in a wonderful variety, can be served hot or cold, eaten as a starter or served as a complete meal. Most are chock full of vitamins and minerals and depending on the ingredients can also be a source of fiber.

Those containing vegetables are also are a good source of phyto-chemicals, the ingredients in plant foods which are thought to protect against disease. Science may not understand all the reasons yet, but what a tasty way to help your health.

Regular chicken and beef broth have been used in the majority of these recipes. If you are concerned about salt or sodium content, choose a reduced sodium broth or make one from scratch when the recipe calls for chicken or beef broth. 35% less salt bouillion envelopes contain about 649 mg of sodium per 1 cup (250 mL) serving as compared with about 900 mg in their regular counterparts.

❖

When tomatoes are in season make this delicious soup. Try using several different types to experiment with a variety of tastes.

◆

This soup can be served hot or cold.

◆

A dollop of light sour cream enhances each soup bowl.

Fresh Tomato Dill Soup

I tbsp	olive oil	15 mL
I tsp	crushed garlic	5 mL
I	medium carrot, chopped	I
I	celery stalk, chopped	I
I cup	chopped onion	250 mL
2 cups	chicken stock	500 mL
5 cups	chopped ripe tomatoes	1.25 L
3 tbsp	tomato paste	45 mL
2 tsp	granulated sugar	10 mL
3 tbsp	chopped fresh dill	45 mL

1. In large nonstick saucepan, heat oil; sauté garlic, carrot, celery and onion until softened, approximately 5 minutes.

2. Add stock, tomatoes and tomato paste; reduce heat, cover and simmer for 20 minutes, stirring occasionally.

3. Purée in food processor until smooth. Add sugar and dill; mix well.

MAKE AHEAD ◆ Prepare and refrigerate early in day, then serve cold or reheat gently.

PER SERVING

1½ ▣ Fruit & Vegetable Choices

½ ▲ Fat & Oil Choice

Calories 106
Carbohydrates . . . . 18 g
Fiber . . . . 4 g
Protein . . . . 3 g
Fat, total . . . . 4 g
Fat, saturated . . . . I g
Sodium . . . . 506 mg
Cholesterol . . . . . . 0 mg

Dill Carrot Soup

This soup can be served hot or cold.

♦

A dollop of yogurt on each bowlful enhances both the appearance and flavor.

♦

Carrots make this soup an excellent source of vitamin A.

1 lb	carrots, sliced (6 to 8 medium)	500 g
2 tsp	vegetable oil	10 mL
2 tsp	crushed garlic	10 mL
1 cup	chopped onion	250 mL
3½ cups	chicken stock	875 mL
¾ cup	2% milk	175 mL
2 tbsp	chopped fresh dill (or 1 tsp [5 mL] dried dillweed)	25 mL
2 tbsp	chopped fresh chives or green onions	25 mL

1. In large saucepan of boiling water, cook carrots just until tender. Drain and return to saucepan; set aside.

2. In nonstick skillet, heat oil; sauté garlic and onion until softened, approximately 5 minutes. Add to carrots along with stock; cover and simmer for 25 minutes.

3. Purée in food processor until smooth, in batches if necessary. Return to saucepan; stir in milk, dill and chives.

MAKE AHEAD ♦ Make and refrigerate up to a day before. If serving warm, reheat gently.

PER SERVING

1	✿ Fruit & Vegetable Choice
½	▲ Fat & Oil Choice

Calories	89
Carbohydrates	13 g
Fiber	2 g
Protein	3 g
Fat, total	3 g
Fat, saturated	1 g
Sodium	863 mg
Cholesterol	2 mg

Preheat broiler

Two baking sheets lined with aluminum foil and sprayed with vegetable spray

TIPS

Regular fresh tomatoes can replace plum.

◆

Dill or coriander can replace basil.

◆

In the summer, grill tomatoes and 2 whole cobs of corn on barbecue.

PER SERVING

½ ■ Starch Choice

1½ ◆ Fruit & Vegetable Choices

½ ◆ Protein Choice

Calories 139
Carbohydrates . . . . 29 g
Fiber . . . . 5 g
Protein . . . . 4 g
Fat, total . . . . 3 g
Fat, saturated . . . . 0 g
Sodium . . . . 216 mg
Cholesterol . . . . . . 0 mg

Roasted Tomato and Corn Soup

2½ lbs	plum tomatoes (about 10)	1.25 kg
1	can (12 oz [341 mL]) corn, drained	1
2 tsp	vegetable oil	10 mL
2 tsp	minced garlic	10 mL
1 cup	chopped onions	250 mL
¾ cup	finely chopped carrots	175 mL
2½ cups	basic vegetable stock (see recipe, page 46)	625 mL
3 tbsp	tomato paste	45 mL
½ cup	chopped fresh basil (or 2 tsp [10 mL] dried)	125 mL

1. Put tomatoes on one baking sheet. With rack 6 inches (15 cm) under broiler, broil tomatoes about 30 minutes, turning occasionally, or until charred on all sides. Meanwhile, spread corn on other baking sheet and broil, stirring occasionally, about 15 minutes or until slightly browned. (Some corn kernels will pop.) When cool enough to handle, chop tomatoes.

2. In a nonstick saucepan, heat oil over medium-high heat. Add garlic, onions and carrots; cook 5 minutes or until softened and beginning to brown. Add roasted tomatoes, stock, tomato paste and, if using, dried basil. (If using fresh basil, wait until Step 3.) Bring to a boil; reduce heat to medium-low, cover and cook 20 minutes or until vegetables tender.

3. In food processor or blender, purée soup. Return to saucepan; stir in corn and, if using, fresh basil.

MAKE AHEAD ◆ Prepare soup up to 2 days in advance, adding more stock, if necessary, when reheating. Freeze up to 4 weeks.

Preheat oven to broil

Baking sheet

Sweet bell peppers and red onions make this a naturally sweet-tasting soup. Sugar may not be necessary.

◆

Start with the lesser amount of stock, adding more to reach the consistency you prefer.

◆

This soup is a very high source of fiber.

Red Onion and Grilled Red Pepper Soup

3	large red bell peppers	3
2 tsp	vegetable oil	10 mL
2 tsp	minced garlic	10 mL
1 tbsp	packed brown sugar	15 mL
5 cups	thinly sliced red onions	1.25 L
3 to 3½ cups	basic vegetable stock (see recipe, page 46)	750 mL to 875 mL

GARNISH

⅓ cup	chopped fresh basil or parsley	75 mL
	Light sour cream (optional)	

1. Arrange oven rack 6 inches (15 cm) under broiler. Cook peppers on baking sheet, turning occasionally, 20 minutes or until charred. Cool. Discard stem, skin and seeds; cut peppers into thin strips. Set aside.

2. In a large nonstick saucepan, heat oil over medium-low heat. Add garlic, brown sugar and red onions; cook, stirring occasionally, 15 minutes or until onions are browned. Stir in stock and red pepper strips; cook 15 minutes longer.

3. In a blender or food processor, purée soup until smooth. Serve hot, garnished with chopped basil or parsley and a dollop of sour cream, if desired.

MAKE AHEAD ◆ Prepare up to 2 days in advance. Add more stock if too thick. Freeze up to 4 weeks.

PER SERVING

2½ ◨ Fruit & Vegetable Choices

½ ✳ Sugar Choice

½ ◉ Protein Choice

½ ▲ Fat & Oil Choice

Calories	187
Carbohydrates	39 g
Fiber	7 g
Protein	5 g
Fat, total	3 g
Fat, saturated	0 g
Sodium	64 mg
Cholesterol	0 mg

This is an unusual, textured, great-tasting soup. A good source of fiber, too.

◆

Replace tarragon with basil, dill, or parsley.

STOCK TIPS

Use vegetable bouillon cubes, powder or canned vegetable bouillon.

◆

Substitute other vegetables of your choice. Try fennel, mushrooms, leeks, potatoes, yams or lettuce.

◆

Freeze in 1 cup (250 mL) portions; label and date.

PER SERVING

1	■ Starch Choice
1	◨ Fruit & Vegetable Choice
½	▲ Fat & Oil Choice

Calories 156
Carbohydrates . . . . 31 g
Fiber . . . . 5 g
Protein . . . . 5 g
Fat, total . . . . 3 g
Fat, saturated . . . . 0 g
Sodium . . . . 112 mg
Cholesterol . . . . . . 0 mg

Artichoke Leek Potato Soup

2 tsp	vegetable oil	10 mL
2 tsp	minced garlic	10 mL
1½ cups	chopped leeks	375 mL
3½ to 4 cups	basic vegetable stock (see recipe, below)	875 mL to 1 L
1½ cups	diced potatoes	375 mL
1 tsp	dried tarragon	5 mL
1	can (14 oz [398 mL]) artichoke hearts, drained and halved	1

1. In a nonstick saucepan, heat oil over medium-low heat. Stir in garlic and leeks, cover and cook 5 minutes.

2. Stir in stock, potatoes, tarragon and artichoke hearts. Bring to a boil; reduce heat to medium-low, cover and cook 15 minutes, or until potato is tender.

3. In a food processor or blender, purée soup.

BASIC VEGETABLE STOCK

8 cups	fresh water or cooking water	2 L
2	stalks celery, chopped	2
2	large onions, chopped	2
2	large carrots, washed and chopped	2
4	cloves garlic, chopped	4
4	bay leaves	4
4	whole cloves (or pinch ground)	4
10	peppercorns, crushed	10
¼ cup	chopped fresh parsley (or ¼ tsp [1 mL] dried)	50 mL
¼ tsp	salt (optional)	1 mL

1. Combine all ingredients in a large pot. Bring to simmer and cook, uncovered, for 45 minutes.

continued on page 47

2. Remove from heat; let cool. Strain, discarding solids. Store in a container with tight-fitting lid. Stock will keep 1 week in refrigerator and several months if frozen.

MAKE AHEAD ◆ Prepare up to 2 days in advance. Freeze up to 4 weeks.

TIPS

Choose the greenest asparagus with straight, firm stalks. The tips should be tightly closed and firm.

◆

This soup can be served warm or cold.

Asparagus and Leek Soup

¾ lb	asparagus	375 g
1½ tsp	vegetable oil	7 mL
1 tsp	crushed garlic	5 mL
1 cup	chopped onion	250 mL
2	leeks, sliced	2
3½ cups	chicken stock	875 mL
1 cup	diced peeled potato	250 mL
	Salt and pepper	
2 tbsp	grated Parmesan cheese	25 mL

1. Trim asparagus; cut stalks into pieces and set tips aside.

2. In large nonstick saucepan, heat oil; sauté garlic, onion, leeks and asparagus stalks just until softened, approximately 10 minutes.

3. Add stock and potato; reduce heat, cover and simmer for 20 to 25 minutes or until vegetables are tender. Purée in food processor until smooth. Taste and adjust seasoning with salt and pepper. Return to saucepan.

4. Steam or microwave reserved asparagus tips just until tender; add to soup. Serve sprinkled with Parmesan cheese.

MAKE AHEAD ◆ Make and refrigerate up to a day before and reheat gently before serving, adding more stock if too thick.

PER SERVING

½ ▪ Starch Choice
1 ▨ Fruit & Vegetable Choice
½ ▨ Protein Choice

Calories 118
Carbohydrates . . . . 20 g
Fiber . . . . 3 g
Protein . . . . 5 g
Fat, total . . . . 3 g
Fat, saturated . . . . 1 g
Sodium . . . . 918 mg
Cholesterol . . . . . . 2 mg

Increase curry to
1½ tsp (7 mL) for more
intense flavor.

◆

This soup is high in fiber
and is an excellent
source of Vitamins A
and C.

◆

Eliminate the ½ ✸
Sugar Choice by using
a granulated sugar
substitute to replace the
honey in this soup. The
carbohydrate content
will be reduced by
almost 7 g/serving.

Curried Broccoli Sweet Potato Soup

2 tsp	vegetable oil	10 mL
1½ tsp	minced garlic	7 mL
1½ cups	chopped onions	375 mL
1 tsp	curry powder	5 mL
4 cups	chicken stock	1 L
4 cups	broccoli florets	1 L
3 cups	peeled, diced sweet potato	750 mL
2 tbsp	honey	25 mL

1. Heat oil in nonstick saucepan over medium heat. Add garlic, onions and curry; cook for 4 minutes or until softened. Add stock, broccoli and sweet potatoes; bring to a boil. Cover, reduce heat to low and simmer for 30 minutes or until vegetables are tender.

2. Transfer soup to food processor or blender; add honey and purée.

MAKE AHEAD ◆ Prepare and refrigerate up to a day ahead and reheat gently before serving, adding more stock if too thick.

PER SERVING

1½ ■ Starch Choices

1 ◢ Fruit & Vegetable Choice

½ ✸ Sugar Choice

½ ▲ Fat & Oil Choice

Calories 216
Carbohydrates . . . . 45 g
Fiber . . . . 6 g
Protein . . . . 5 g
Fat, total . . . . 3 g
Fat, saturated . . . . 0 g
Sodium . . . . 971 mg
Cholesterol . . . . . . 0 mg

Creamy Salmon Dill Bisque

6 oz	salmon fillet	150 g
2 tsp	margarine or butter	10 mL
1 tsp	minced garlic	5 mL
1 cup	chopped onions	250 mL
1 cup	chopped carrots	250 mL
½ cup	chopped celery	125 mL
1 tbsp	tomato paste	15 mL
2¼ cups	chicken stock	550 mL
1½ cups	peeled, chopped potatoes	375 mL
½ cup	2% milk	125 mL
¼ cup	chopped fresh dill	50 mL

1. In nonstick pan sprayed with vegetable spray, cook salmon over high heat for 3 minutes, then turn and cook 2 minutes longer, or until just barely done at center. Set aside.

2. Melt margarine in nonstick saucepan sprayed with vegetable spray over medium heat. Add garlic, onions, carrots, and celery; cook for 5 minutes or until onion is softened. Add tomato paste, stock and potatoes; bring to a boil. Cover, reduce heat to low and simmer for 20 minutes or until carrots and potatoes are tender.

3. Transfer soup to food processor or blender and purée. Return to saucepan and stir in milk and dill. Flake the cooked salmon. Add to soup and serve.

MAKE AHEAD ◆ Prepare up to a day ahead, but do not add salmon until just ready to serve. Add more stock if soup is too thick.

A dollop of light sour cream on top of each bowlful gives a great taste and sophisticated look.

◆

Unlike traditional broccoli soups, this soup contains lentils, which help make it an excellent source of folate. This soup is an excellent source of vitamin A and good source of magnesium, iron and vitamin C.

Broccoli and Lentil Soup

1½ tsp	vegetable oil	7 mL
2 tsp	crushed garlic	10 mL
1	medium onion, chopped	1
1	celery stalk, chopped	1
1	large carrot, chopped	1
4 cups	chicken stock	1 L
2½ cups	chopped broccoli	625 mL
¾ cup	dried green lentils	175 mL
2 tbsp	grated Parmesan cheese	25 mL

1. In large nonstick saucepan, heat oil; sauté garlic, onion, celery and carrot until softened, approximately 5 minutes.

2. Add stock, broccoli and lentils; cover and simmer for 30 minutes, stirring occasionally, or until lentils are tender.

3. Purée in food processor until creamy and smooth. Serve sprinkled with Parmesan.

MAKE AHEAD ◆ Prepare and refrigerate up to a day before and reheat gently, adding more stock if too thick.

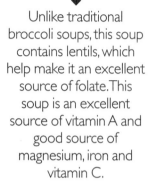

PER SERVING

1	■ Starch Choice
1	⬤ Protein Choice

Calories 139
Carbohydrates . . . . 20 g
Fiber . . . . 4 g
Protein . . . . 10 g
Fat, total . . . . 3 g
Fat, saturated . . . . 1 g
Sodium . . . . 999 mg
Cholesterol . . . . . . 2 mg

Oyster or cremini mushrooms are the best to use here. If unavailable, substitute white common mushrooms.

◆

Barley is available in "pearl" and "pot" varieties; whichever you use, cook until tender.

◆

This soup is a good source of fiber.

◆

Use some dried mushrooms to really highlight this dish.

Wild Mushroom and Barley Soup

2 tsp	vegetable oil	10 mL
2 tsp	minced garlic	10 mL
1 cup	chopped onions	250 mL
3½ cups	basic vegetable stock (see recipe, page 46)	875 mL
1 can	(19 oz [540 mL]) tomatoes, crushed	1
½ cup	barley	125 mL
½ tsp	dried thyme	2 mL
¼ tsp	freshly ground black pepper	1 mL
8 oz	wild mushrooms, sliced (see Tip, at left)	250 g

1. In a nonstick saucepan, heat oil over medium heat. Add garlic and onions; cook 4 minutes or until softened.

2. Stir in stock, tomatoes, barley, thyme and pepper. Bring to a boil; reduce heat to medium-low, cover and simmer 40 to 50 minutes, or until barley is tender.

3. Meanwhile, in a nonstick frying pan sprayed with vegetable spray, cook mushrooms over high heat, stirring, 8 minutes or until browned.

4. Stir mushrooms into soup and serve.

MAKE AHEAD ◆ Prepare up to 2 days in advance. Add more stock when reheating if too thick. Freeze for up to 3 weeks.

PER SERVING

1	■	Starch Choice
1	◢	Fruit & Vegetable Choice
½	▲	Fat & Oil Choice

Calories 135
Carbohydrates . . . . 28 g
Fiber . . . . 4 g
Protein . . . . 4 g
Fat, total . . . . 2 g
Fat, saturated . . . . 0 g
Sodium . . . . 289 mg
Cholesterol . . . . . . 0 mg

Use either pot or pearl barley.

◆

Common mushrooms should be firm and dry to the touch. They are very perishable and should be cooked within 48 hours.

◆

Add a chunk of low-fat cheese, low-fat milk, ½ cup (125 mL) of unsweetened applesauce and cinnamon snap cookies for a delicious complete lunch.

Vegetable Beef Barley Soup

1 tbsp	vegetable oil	15 mL
2 tsp	crushed garlic	10 mL
1	medium onion, diced	1
2	celery stalks, diced	2
2	carrots, diced	2
2 cups	sliced mushrooms	500 mL
3½ cups	(approx) beef stock	875 mL
⅓ cup	barley	75 mL
2	small potatoes, peeled and diced	2
4 oz	stewing beef, diced	125 g
2 tbsp	chopped fresh parsley	25 mL

1. In large nonstick saucepan, heat oil; sauté garlic, onion, celery, carrots and mushrooms until tender, approximately 10 minutes.

2. Add stock, barley, potatoes and beef; cover, reduce heat and simmer approximately 50 minutes or until barley and potatoes are tender, stirring occasionally.

MAKE AHEAD ◆ Make and refrigerate up to a day before. Reheat gently just before serving, adding more stock if too thick.

PER SERVING

1½ ■ Starch Choices

½ ◆ Fruit & Vegetable Choice

1 ◉ Protein Choice

½ ▲ Fat & Oil Choice

Calories 208

Carbohydrates . . . . 31 g

Fiber . . . . 4 g

Protein . . . . 11 g

Fat, total . . . . 5 g

Fat, saturated . . . . 1 g

Sodium . . . . 1009 mg

Cholesterol . . . . . 13 mg

Frozen corn niblets would be fine to use. If time is available, make your own stock for a really delicious chowder.

◆

Corn and potatoes are two vegetables which the "Good Health Eating Guide" considers ■ Starch choices.

Potato Corn Chowder

2 cups	corn niblets (canned or fresh)	500 mL
1 ½ tsp	margarine	7 mL
1 cup	chopped onions	250 mL
½ cup	chopped sweet red pepper	125 mL
1 tsp	crushed garlic	5 mL
1 cup	diced peeled potato	250 mL
1 ⅓ cups	chicken stock	325 mL
2 tbsp	all-purpose flour	25 mL
1 ½ cups	2% milk	375 mL
¼ tsp	Worcestershire sauce	1 mL
	Pepper	

1. In food processor, process 1 cup (250 mL) of the corn until puréed; add to remaining corn and set aside.

2. In large nonstick saucepan, melt margarine; sauté onions, red pepper and garlic for 5 minutes. Add potato and stock; simmer, covered, until potato is tender, approximately 15 minutes.

3. Add corn mixture to soup; cook for 5 minutes. Stir in flour and cook for 1 minute. Add milk, Worcestershire sauce, and pepper to taste; cook on medium heat for approximately 5 minutes or just until thickened.

MAKE AHEAD ◆ Make and refrigerate early in day and reheat gently, adding more stock or milk if too thick.

PER SERVING

1 ½ ■ Starch Choices
½ ◆ 2% Milk Choice
½ ▲ Fat & Oil Choice
1 ◆◆ Extra Choice

Calories 176
Carbohydrates . . . . 32 g
Fiber . . . . 4 g
Protein . . . . 7 g
Fat, total . . . . 4 g
Fat, saturated . . . . 1 g
Sodium . . . . 441 mg
Cholesterol . . . . . . 6 mg

Sweet potatoes are a nice substitute for white potatoes. The soup acquires a sweeter taste.

◆

This soup is an excellent source of iron, vitamins A, C, niacin and B_{12}.

Clam and Pasta Chowder

2 tsp	vegetable oil	10 mL
1 ½ tsp	crushed garlic	7 mL
1 cup	chopped onions	250 mL
½ cup	finely chopped carrots	125 mL
⅔ cup	chopped sweet green peppers	150 mL
1 ½	cans (5 oz [140 mL]) clams, reserving juice from 1 can	1 ½
1 cup	diced potatoes	250 mL
2 ½ cups	canned or fresh tomatoes, crushed	625 mL
2 ½ cups	seafood or chicken stock	625 mL
⅓ cup	tubetti or macaroni	75 mL

1. In large nonstick saucepan, heat oil; sauté garlic, onions, carrots and green peppers until tender, approximately 5 minutes.

2. Add juice of 1 can of clams, potatoes, tomatoes and stock. Cover and simmer for 20 minutes.

3. Add reserved clams and tubetti. Simmer for 10 minutes or until pasta is cooked.

MAKE AHEAD ◆ Prepare early in day, not adding pasta until 10 minutes before serving.

PER SERVING

½ ▦ Starch Choice

1 ½ ◗ Fruit & Vegetable Choices

1 ◗ Protein Choice

Calories 149
Carbohydrates . . . . 24 g
Fiber . . . . 3 g
Protein . . . . 8 g
Fat, total . . . . 3 g
Fat, saturated . . . . 0 g
Sodium . . . . 643 mg
Cholesterol . . . . . 12 mg

Ground pork or veal can replace chicken.

◆

Sweet potatoes are a nice change from white potatoes.

◆

Adjust spiciness by adding more cayenne.

◆

Canned tomatoes and chicken stock are both sources of salt or sodium in this recipe. Reduce sodium by using low sodium chicken broth. Almost a "meal in a bowl", finish with fresh fruit and low-fat milk.

Chili, Chicken, Bean and Pasta Stew

2 tsp	vegetable oil	10 mL
2 tsp	crushed garlic	10 mL
1 cup	chopped onions	250 mL
8 oz	ground chicken	250 g
1	can (19 oz [540 mL]) crushed tomatoes	1
2½ cups	chicken stock	625 mL
1½ cups	diced peeled potatoes	375 mL
½ cup	canned red kidney beans, drained	125 mL
½ cup	canned chick peas, drained	125 mL
2 tbsp	tomato paste	25 mL
1 tbsp	chili powder	15 mL
2 tsp	dried basil	10 mL
1 tsp	dried oregano	5 mL
Pinch	cayenne	Pinch
⅓ cup	macaroni	75 mL

1. In large nonstick saucepan, heat oil; sauté garlic and onions until softened, approximately 5 minutes.

2. Add chicken and cook, stirring to break up chunks, until no longer pink; pour off any fat.

3. Add tomatoes, stock, potatoes, kidney beans, chick peas, tomato paste, chili powder, basil, oregano and cayenne. Cover and reduce heat; simmer for 40 minutes, stirring occasionally.

4. Add pasta; cook until firm to the bite, approximately 10 minutes.

MAKE AHEAD ◆ Prepare soup up to a day ahead. Add pasta until 10 minutes before serving.

PER SERVING

1½ ■ Starch Choices

½ ◢ Fruit & Vegetable Choice

1½ ◨ Protein Choices

1 ▲ Fat & Oil Choice

1 ✦✦ Extra Choice

Calories 267
Carbohydrates . . . . 36 g
Fiber . . . . 3 g
Protein . . . . 14 g
Fat, total . . . . 9 g
Fat, saturated . . . . 0 g
Sodium . . . . 1001 mg
Cholesterol . . . . . . 0 mg

Try to ensure that mango is ripe. They can be stored in the refrigerator for up to 3 days. How can you tell if a mango is ripe? It should have a strong fragrance and feel slightly soft if you apply gentle pressure.

◆

This soup can also be served at room temperature.

Cold Mango Soup

2 tsp	vegetable oil	10 mL
½ cup	chopped onions	125 mL
2 tsp	minced garlic	10 mL
2 cups	basic vegetable stock (see recipe, page 46)	500 mL
2½ cups	chopped ripe mango (about 2 large)	625 mL

GARNISH (OPTIONAL)
2% plain yogurt
Coriander leaves

1. In a nonstick saucepan, heat oil over medium heat. Add onions and garlic; cook, stirring, 4 minutes or until browned.

2. Add stock. Bring to a boil; reduce heat to medium-low and cook 5 minutes or until onions are soft.

3. Transfer mixture to a food processor. Add 2 cups (500 mL) of the mango. Purée until smooth. Stir in remaining chopped mango.

4. Chill 2 hours or until cold. Serve with a dollop of yogurt and garnish with coriander, if desired.

MAKE AHEAD ◆ Prepare up to 2 days in advance. Freeze up to 3 weeks.

PER SERVING

2 ▮ Fruit & Vegetable Choices

½ ▲ Fat & Oil Choice

Calories	110
Carbohydrates	23 g
Fiber	3 g
Protein	1 g
Fat, total	3 g
Fat, saturated	0 g
Sodium	38 mg
Cholesterol	0 mg

Salads

Salads can serve as a starter, act as a side dish or be a complete meal. The combination of ingredients can provide delicious taste, texture and variety.

People attempting to increase their intake of fresh vegetables may include traditional "salads" such as coleslaw more often, failing to consider commercial dressings, sweet sauces or brines used in their preparation. Choose salad ingredients wisely and pay attention to how they "fit" into your meal plan. Use some of the delicious salads which follow to increase your meal time flexibility, provide great lunch time alternatives and pack away plenty of good nutrition at the same time.

❖

Sweet fruit and a combination of lettuces make this a perfect salad.

◆

If you don't care for the bitter flavor of curly endive and radicchio, use romaine or Bibb lettuce instead.

◆

If you don't want the salad to wilt, use a larger amount of romaine lettuce.

Pear, Lettuce and Feta Cheese Salad

DRESSING

2 tbsp	raspberry vinegar	25 mL
2 ½ tbsp	olive oil	35 mL
1 tsp	minced garlic	5 mL
1 ½ tsp	honey	7 mL
1 tsp	sesame oil	5 mL

SALAD

4 cups	red or green leaf lettuce, washed, dried and torn into pieces	1 L
1 ½ cups	curly endive or escarole, washed, dried and torn into pieces	375 mL
1 ½ cups	radicchio, washed, dried and torn into pieces	375 mL
1 cup	diced pears (about 1 pear)	250 mL
2 oz	feta cheese, crumbled	50 g
⅓ cup	sliced black olives	75 mL

1. Prepare the dressing: In a small bowl, whisk together vinegar, olive oil, garlic, honey and sesame oil; set aside.

2. Make the salad: In a serving bowl, combine leaf lettuce, curly endive, radicchio, pears, feta and olives. Pour dressing over; toss gently to coat. Serve immediately.

MAKE AHEAD ◆ Prepare salad and dressing early in the day. Toss just before serving.

PER SERVING

1	🍃 Fruit & Vegetable Choice
2	▲ Fat & Oil Choices

Calories	128
Carbohydrates	10 g
Fiber	2 g
Protein	3 g
Fat, total	9 g
Fat, saturated	2 g
Sodium	144 mg
Cholesterol	9 mg

Four-Tomato Salad

½ cup	sun-dried tomatoes	125 mL
2 cups	sliced field tomatoes	500 mL
2 cups	halved red or yellow cherry tomatoes	500 mL
2 cups	quartered plum tomatoes	500 mL
I cup	sliced red onions	250 mL

DRESSING

3 tbsp	olive oil	45 mL
¼ cup	balsamic vinegar	50 mL
I ½ tsp	minced garlic	7 mL
½ cup	chopped fresh basil (or 2 tsp [10 mL] dried)	125 mL
⅛ tsp	ground black pepper	0.5 mL

1. Pour boiling water over sun-dried tomatoes. Let rest for 15 minutes until softened. Drain and slice.

2. Place sun-dried tomatoes, field tomatoes, cherry tomatoes, plum tomatoes, red onions and fresh basil in serving bowl or on platter.

3. Whisk together olive oil, balsamic vinegar, garlic and pepper; pour over tomatoes just before serving.

MAKE AHEAD ◆ Prepare dressing early in the day only if using dried basil. Salad portion can be prepared early in the day.

Any combination of tomatoes can be used if those specified here are not available.

◆

Yellow, larger tomatoes, if available, are great to add.

◆

Removing seeds from field tomatoes will eliminate excess liquid.

◆

Do not toss this salad until just ready to serve.

◆

This recipe is an excellent source of vitamin C, good source of magnesium and folate, and is packed with lycopene (a phytochemical).

PER SERVING

1½ 🍃 Fruit & Vegetable Choices

1½ ▲ Fat & Oil Choices

Calories 134
Carbohydrates . . . . 17 g
Fiber . . . . 3 g
Protein . . . . 3 g
Fat, total . . . . 8 g
Fat, saturated . . . . I g
Sodium . . . . 116 mg
Cholesterol . . . . . . 0 mg

A combination of
red and white cabbage
is attractive.

◆

For curry lovers, 1 tsp
(5 mL) curry powder
can be added to
the dressing.

Creamy Coleslaw
with Apples and Raisins

1	medium carrot, diced	1
1/3 cup	finely chopped red onion	75 mL
1/2 cup	finely chopped sweet red or green pepper	125 mL
2	green onions, diced	2
3 cups	thinly sliced white or red cabbage	750 mL
1/3 cup	diced (unpeeled) apple	75 mL
1/3 cup	raisins	75 mL
DRESSING		
1/4 cup	light mayonnaise	50 mL
2 tbsp	2% yogurt	25 mL
2 tbsp	lemon juice	25 mL
1 1/2 tsp	honey	7 mL
	Salt and pepper	

1. In serving bowl, combine carrot, red onion, red pepper, green onions, cabbage, apple and raisins.

2. Dressing: In small bowl, stir together mayonnaise, yogurt, lemon juice, honey, and salt and pepper to taste, mixing well. Pour over salad and toss gently to combine.

MAKE AHEAD ◆ Prepare and refrigerate early in day and stir well before serving.

PER SERVING

2½ ◱ Fruit & Vegetable Choices

1 ▲ Fat & Oil Choice

Calories 147
Carbohydrates . . . . 26 g
Fiber . . . . 3 g
Protein . . . . 2 g
Fat, total . . . . 5 g
Fat, saturated . . . . 1 g
Sodium . . . . 179 mg
Cholesterol . . . . . . 3 mg

TIP

Toast sesame seeds in nonstick skillet over high heat for 2 to 3 minutes.

Oriental Vegetable Salad

2½ cups	trimmed green beans	625 mL
2 cups	asparagus cut into 1-inch (2.5 cm) pieces	500 mL
1½ cups	halved snow peas	375 mL
1¾ cups	bean sprouts	425 mL
1½ cups	sliced red bell peppers	375 mL
1 cup	chopped baby corn cobs	250 mL
¾ cup	canned sliced water chestnuts, drained	175 mL
¾ cup	canned mandarin oranges, drained	175 mL

DRESSING

4 tsp	soya sauce	20 mL
4 tsp	rice wine vinegar	20 mL
1 tbsp	olive oil	15 mL
1 tbsp	honey	15 mL
2 tsp	sesame oil	10 mL
2 tsp	toasted sesame seeds	10 mL
1½ tsp	minced garlic	7 mL
1 tsp	minced gingerroot	5 mL

1. Boil or steam green beans and asparagus for 2 to 3 minutes or until tender-crisp; drain. Rinse under cold water and drain; transfer to a large serving bowl.

2. Boil or steam snow peas 45 seconds or until tender-crisp; drain. Rinse under cold water and drain; add to serving bowl along with bean sprouts, red peppers, corn cobs, water chestnuts and mandarin oranges. Toss to combine.

3. In a small bowl, whisk together soya sauce, vinegar, olive oil, honey, sesame oil, sesame seeds, garlic and ginger. Pour over salad; toss to coat.

MAKE AHEAD ◆ Prepare salad and dressing earlier in the day. Keep separate in refrigerator until ready to serve.

Any combination of
seafood is good, but
these three work
very well.

◆

Try fresh coriander
or Italian parsley instead
of the dill.

◆

This salad can be served
as a lunch item with a
multigrain bagel and
low-fat milk. Fresh fruit
can finish the meal.

Seafood Salad
with Dill Dressing

4 oz	deveined peeled (uncooked) shrimp, chopped	125 g
4 oz	scallops, chopped	125 g
4 oz	squid, chopped	125 g
½ cup	chopped sweet red or yellow pepper	125 mL
½ cup	chopped sweet green pepper	125 mL
½ cup	chopped celery	125 mL
½ cup	chopped red onion	125 mL
1	large green onion, sliced	1
	Lettuce leaves	
	Parsley sprigs	

DRESSING

½ cup	2% yogurt	125 mL
2 tbsp	light mayonnaise	25 mL
3 tbsp	chopped fresh parsley	45 mL
¼ cup	chopped fresh dill (or 4 tsp [20 mL] dried dillweed)	50 mL
1 tsp	Dijon mustard	5 mL
1 tsp	crushed garlic	5 mL
	Salt and pepper	

1. In shallow saucepan, bring 2 cups (500 mL) water to boil; reduce heat to simmer. Add shrimp, scallops and squid; cover and poach until shrimp are pink and squid and scallops opaque, approximately 2 minutes. Drain and rinse with cold water; drain well and place in bowl. Add red and green peppers, celery and red and green onions.

2. Dressing: In small bowl, combine yogurt, mayonnaise, parsley, dill, mustard, garlic, and salt and pepper to taste, mixing well. Pour over salad and toss well.

continued on page 63

PER SERVING

1 ◢ Fruit & Vegetable Choice

2½ ◢ Protein Choices

Calories 169
Carbohydrates . . . . 12 g
Fiber . . . . 2 g
Protein . . . . 19 g
Fat, total . . . . 5 g
Fat, saturated . . . . 1 g
Sodium . . . . 289 mg
Cholesterol . . . . 135 mg

3. Line serving bowl with lettuce; top with salad and garnish with parsley.

MAKE AHEAD ◆ Prepare and refrigerate salad and dressing early in day, but do not combine until 2 hours before eating. Stir just before serving.

❖

TIP

To make your own croutons, mix 1 tsp (5 mL) each crushed garlic and melted margarine; brush on both sides of 1 slice whole wheat bread. Broil for 3 minutes until browned, then cut into cubes.

Caesar Salad
with Baby Shrimp

2 oz	cooked baby shrimp	50 g
1	medium head romaine lettuce, torn into bite-sized pieces	1
1 tbsp	grated Parmesan cheese	15 mL
1 cup	croutons, preferably homemade	250 mL

DRESSING

1	egg	1
1 tsp	crushed garlic	5 mL
1	anchovy, minced	1
4 tsp	lemon juice	20 mL
1 tbsp	red wine vinegar	15 mL
1 tsp	Dijon mustard	5 mL
1 tbsp	grated Parmesan cheese	15 mL
2 tbsp	olive oil	25 mL

1. In large bowl, place shrimp, lettuce, cheese and croutons.

2. Dressing: In small bowl, combine egg, garlic, anchovy, lemon juice, vinegar, mustard and cheese; gradually whisk in oil until combined. Pour over salad and toss to coat.

MAKE AHEAD ◆ Dressing can be prepared and refrigerated early in the day; toss with salad just before serving.

PER SERVING

½ ✿ Fruit & Vegetable Choice

½ ✿ Protein Choice

1 ▲ Fat & Oil Choice

Calories 99
Carbohydrates . . . . . 5 g
Fiber . . . . 1 g
Protein . . . . 5 g
Fat, total . . . . 7 g
Fat, saturated . . . . 1 g
Sodium . . . . 117 mg
Cholesterol . . . . . 56 mg

TIPS

Orzo is a rice-shaped pasta. If unavailable, substitute a small shell pasta.

◆

Substitute squid or any firm white fish for part or all of the shrimp or scallops.

◆

Definitely use fresh lemon juice — bottled will give too tart a taste. If a less intense lemon flavor is desired, use 3 tbsp (45 mL) instead of ¼ cup (50 mL).

Greek Orzo Seafood Salad

1¾ cups	orzo	425 mL
8 oz	shrimp or scallops or a combination, chopped	250 g
1 cup	halved snow peas	250 mL
12 oz	tomatoes, chopped	375 g
3 oz	feta cheese, crumbled	75 g

DRESSING

¼ cup	olive oil	50 mL
¼ cup	freshly squeezed lemon juice	50 mL
1 tbsp	dried oregano (or ⅓ cup [75 mL] chopped fresh)	15 mL
2 tsp	minced garlic	10 mL
2 tsp	grated lemon zest	10 mL
¼ tsp	ground black pepper	1 mL

1. In large pot of boiling water cook the orzo for 8 to 10 minutes or until tender but firm; rinse under cold water and drain. Put in large serving bowl.

2. In nonstick skillet sprayed with vegetable spray, cook shrimp or scallops over high heat for 2 minutes or until just done at center. Drain any excess liquid. Add to orzo in serving bowl.

3. In a saucepan of boiling water, blanch snow peas for 1 minute, or until tender-crisp; refresh in cold water and drain. Place in serving bowl, along with tomatoes and feta cheese.

4. In small bowl whisk together olive oil, lemon juice, oregano, garlic, lemon zest and pepper; pour over salad and toss well. Chill before serving.

MAKE AHEAD ◆ Prepare early in the day and keep refrigerated. This tastes fine the next day.

PER SERVING

1	■ Starch Choice
½	● Fruit & Vegetable Choice
1	● Protein Choice
1½	▲ Fat & Oil Choices

Calories	226
Carbohydrates	23 g
Fiber	2 g
Protein	11 g
Fat, total	10 g
Fat, saturated	3 g
Sodium	163 mg
Cholesterol	53 mg

Pesto Potato Salad (page 70) ➤
Overleaf: Swordfish with
Mango Coriander Salsa (page 79)

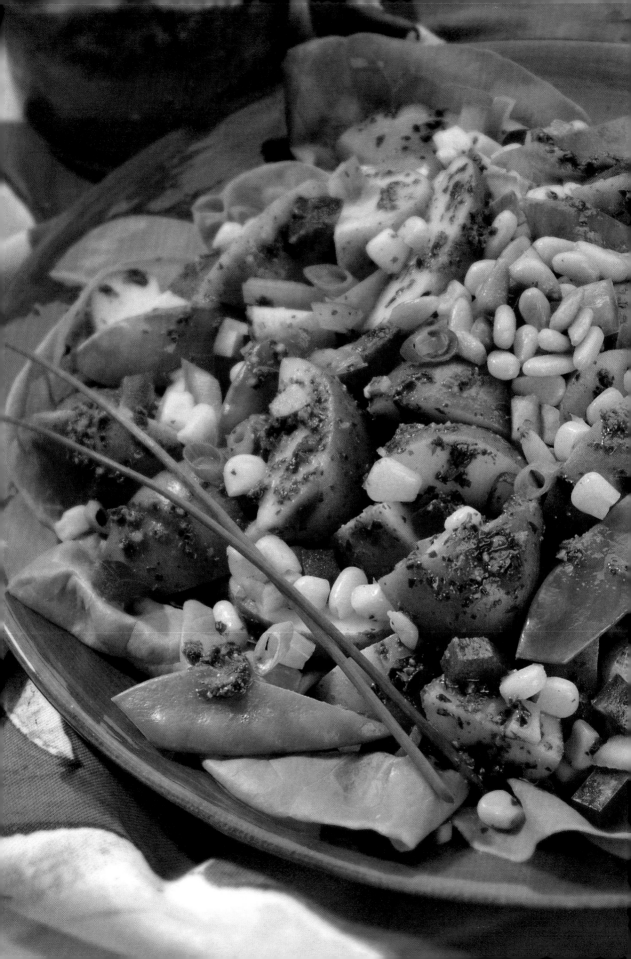

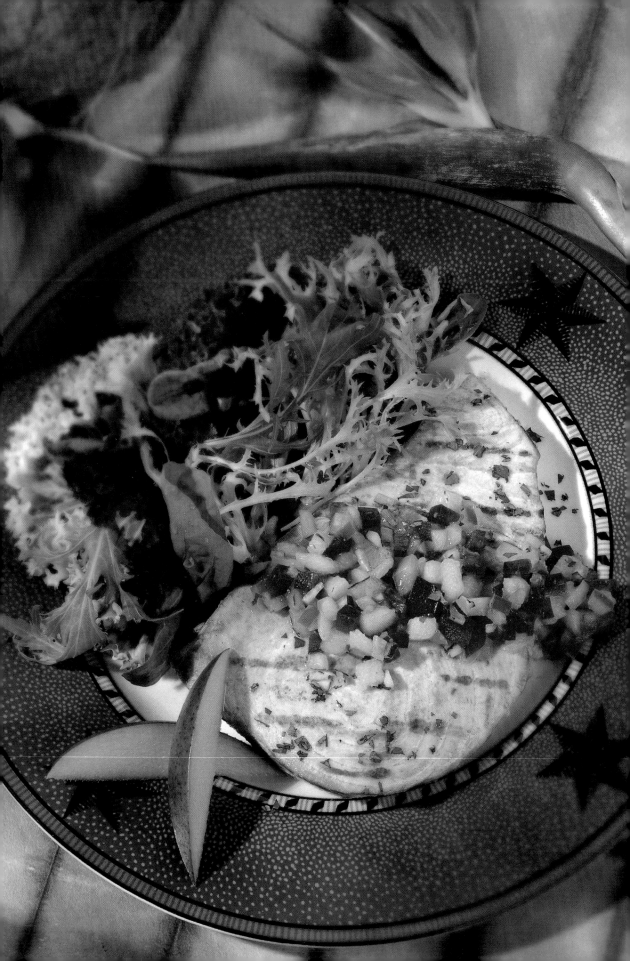

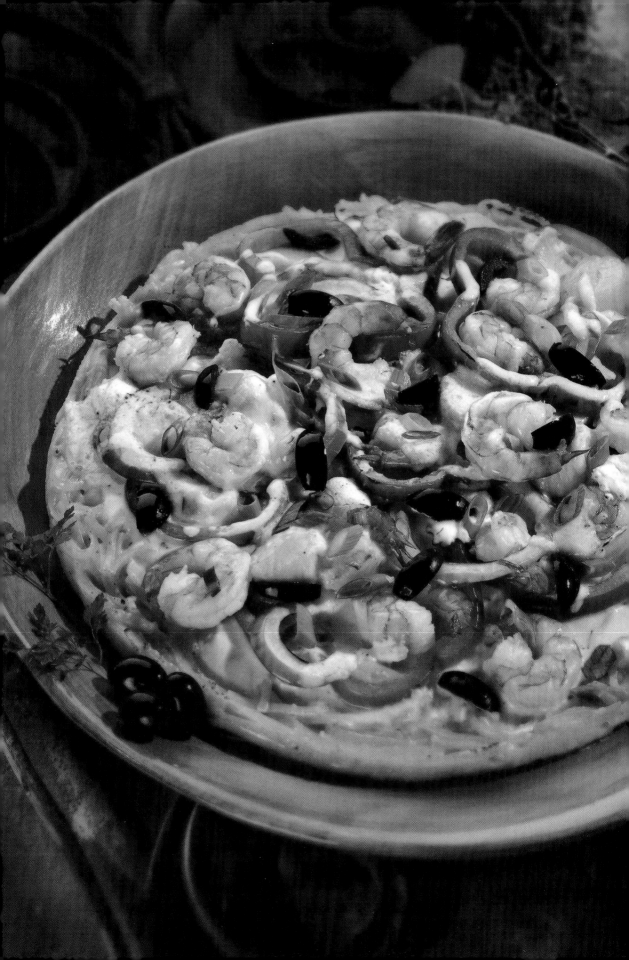

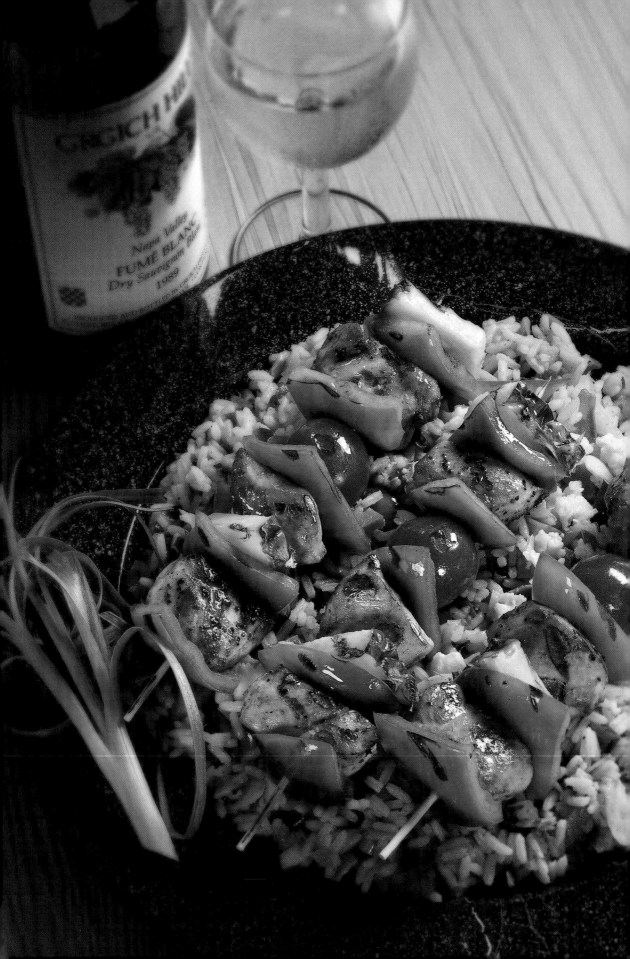

If tarragon is unavailable, substitute ¼ cup (50 mL) chopped fresh dill.

◆

Fresh tuna or swordfish are delicious substitutes for chicken.

◆

Toast pecans in small skillet on medium heat until browned, 2 to 3 minutes.

PER SERVING

1½ ▣ Fruit & Vegetable Choices

3½ ▣ Protein Choices

Calories 179
Carbohydrates . . . . 17 g
Fiber . . . . 4 g
Protein . . . . 17 g
Fat, total . . . . 6 g
Fat, saturated . . . . 1 g
Sodium . . . . 164 mg
Cholesterol . . . . . 35 mg

Chicken Salad
with Tarragon and Pecans

10 oz	boneless skinless chicken breast, cubed	300 g
¾ cup	chopped sweet red or green pepper	175 mL
¾ cup	chopped carrot	175 mL
¾ cup	chopped broccoli florets	175 mL
¾ cup	chopped snow peas	175 mL
¾ cup	chopped red onion	175 mL
1 tbsp	chopped pecans, toasted	15 mL

DRESSING

½ cup	2% yogurt	125 mL
2 tbsp	lemon juice	25 mL
2 tbsp	light mayonnaise	25 mL
1 tsp	crushed garlic	5 mL
1 tsp	Dijon mustard	5 mL
¼ cup	chopped fresh parsley	50 mL
2 tsp	dried tarragon (or 3 tbsp [45 mL] chopped fresh)	10 mL
	Salt and pepper	

1. In small saucepan, bring 2 cups (500 mL) water to boil; reduce heat to simmer. Add chicken; cover and cook just until no longer pink inside, 2 to 4 minutes. Drain and place in serving bowl.

2. Add red pepper, carrot, broccoli, snow peas and onion; toss well.

3. Dressing: In small bowl, combine yogurt, lemon juice, mayonnaise, garlic, mustard, parsley, tarragon, and salt and pepper to taste; pour over chicken and mix well. Taste and adjust seasoning. Sprinkle with pecans.

MAKE AHEAD ◆ Prepare and refrigerate salad and dressing separately early in day, but do not mix until ready to serve.

≺ Chicken Kabobs with Ginger Lemon Marinade (page 91)
Overleaf: Seafood Pasta Pizza with Dill and Goat Cheese (page 84)

This recipe can be
prepared using all wild
rice or all white rice.

◆

Great salad for brunch
or picnic. Sits well
for hours.

Polynesian Wild Rice Salad

2 cups	chicken stock	500 mL
½ cup	white rice	125 mL
½ cup	wild rice	125 mL
1 cup	halved snow peas	250 mL
1 cup	chopped red peppers	250 mL
¾ cup	chopped celery	175 mL
⅔ cup	sliced water chestnuts	150 mL
½ cup	canned mandarin oranges, drained	125 mL
2	medium green onions, chopped	2

DRESSING

2 tsp	orange juice concentrate, thawed	10 mL
2 tsp	honey	10 mL
1 tsp	soya sauce	5 mL
1 tsp	vegetable oil	5 mL
½ tsp	sesame oil	2 mL
½ tsp	lemon juice	2 mL
½ tsp	minced garlic	2 mL
¼ tsp	minced gingerroot	1 mL

1. Bring stock to boil in medium saucepan; add wild rice and white rice. Cover, reduce heat to medium low and simmer for 15 to 20 minutes, or until rice is tender and liquid is absorbed. Rinse with cold water. Put rice in serving bowl.

2. In a saucepan of boiling water or microwave, blanch snow peas for 1 or 2 minutes or until tender-crisp; refresh in cold water and drain. Add to serving bowl along with red peppers, celery, water chestnuts, mandarin oranges and green onions; toss well.

continued on page 67

PER SERVING

1	■ Starch Choice
1½	◗ Fruit & Vegetable Choices
½	▲ Fat & Oil Choice

Calories 157
Carbohydrates . . . . 32 g
Fiber . . . . 3 g
Protein . . . . 5 g
Fat, total . . . . 2 g
Fat, saturated . . . . 0 g
Sodium . . . . 552 mg
Cholesterol . . . . . . 0 mg

3. In small bowl, whisk together orange juice concentrate, honey, soya sauce, vegetable oil, sesame oil, lemon juice, garlic and ginger; pour over salad and toss well.

MAKE AHEAD ◆ Prepare up to a day ahead. Keep refrigerated and stir well before serving.

❖

Serves 6 to 8
as an appetizer

TIPS

This recipe needs little oil because the tomatoes give it the necessary liquid. Use ripe juicy tomatoes.

◆

Sweet Vidalia onions are great to use in season.

◆

If your meal plan calls for extra protein add additional Brie.

PER SERVING

2	■	Starch Choices
½	◗	Fruit & Vegetable Choice
½	◉	Protein Choice
1½	▲	Fat & Oil Choices
1	✦✦	Extra Choice

Calories 274
Carbohydrates . . . . 40 g
Fiber . . . . 3 g
Protein . . . . 9 g
Fat, total . . . . 9 g
Fat, saturated . . . . 3 g
Sodium . . . . 94 mg
Cholesterol . . . . . 11 mg

Penne with Brie Cheese, Tomatoes and Basil

12 oz	penne	375 g
1 ½ lb	chopped tomatoes	750 g
2 tsp	crushed garlic	10 mL
1 cup	chopped red onions	250 mL
3 oz	diced Brie cheese	75 g
⅓ cup	sliced black olives	75 mL
⅔ cup	chopped fresh basil (or 2 tsp [10 mL] dried)	150 mL
3 tbsp	olive oil	45 mL
2 tbsp	lemon juice	25 mL
1 tbsp	red wine vinegar	15 mL
	Pepper	

1. Cook pasta in boiling water according to package instructions or until firm to the bite. Rinse with cold water. Drain and place in serving bowl.

2. Add tomatoes, garlic, onions, cheese, olives, basil, oil, lemon juice, vinegar and pepper. Mix well.

MAKE AHEAD ◆ Prepare tomato dressing early in day and let marinate. Do not toss until ready to serve.

Bulgur wheat can often be found in grocery stores next to the rice and other grains. If not, health food stores always carry it.

◆

A granular sugar substitute can replace the honey in this recipe and eliminate the ½ ✱ Sugar choice or save about 5 g of carbohydrate/serving.

Asian Tabbouleh Salad with Soya Orange Dressing

SALAD

2 cups	basic vegetable stock (see recipe, page 46) or water	500 mL
1½ cups	bulgur wheat	375 mL
1 cup	finely chopped red bell peppers	250 mL
1 cup	finely chopped water chestnuts	250 mL
½ cup	finely chopped green onions	125 mL
⅓ cup	chopped fresh coriander	75 mL
1 cup	broccoli florets	250 mL
1 cup	chopped snow peas	250 mL

DRESSING

4 tsp	orange juice concentrate	20 mL
4 tsp	honey	20 mL
2½ tsp	sesame oil	12 mL
2½ tsp	soya sauce	12 mL
1 tsp	minced garlic	5 mL
1 tsp	freshly squeezed lemon juice	5 mL
¾ tsp	minced gingerroot	4 mL

1. In a saucepan bring stock or water to a boil. Stir in bulgur, cover and turn heat off. Let stand 15 minutes; drain, rinse with cold water and place in a serving bowl. Stir in red peppers, water chestnuts, green onions and coriander.

2. Boil or steam broccoli florets and snow peas 2 minutes or until tender-crisp. Rinse under cold water, drain and add to bulgur mixture.

continued on page 69

PER SERVING

1½ ▣ Starch Choices

1 ◐ Fruit & Vegetable Choices

½ ✱ Sugar Choice

½ ◉ Protein Choice

Calories 217
Carbohydrates . . . . 45 g
Fiber . . . . 6 g
Protein . . . . 7 g
Fat, total . . . . 3 g
Fat, saturated . . . . 0 g
Sodium . . . . 177 mg
Cholesterol . . . . . . 0 mg

3. Make the dressing: In a small bowl, whisk together orange juice concentrate, honey, sesame oil, soya sauce, garlic, lemon juice and ginger. Pour over bulgur mixture and toss to coat. Serve chilled or at room temperature.

MAKE AHEAD ◆ Prepare early in the day. Dressing can be poured over early, allowing salad to marinate.

Pasta Salad with Apricots, Dates and Orange Dressing

12 oz	medium shell pasta	375 g
1 ½ cups	diced sweet red or green peppers	375 mL
¾ cup	diced dried apricots	175 mL
¾ cup	diced dried dates	175 mL
½ cup	chopped green onions	125 mL

DRESSING

3 tbsp	balsamic vinegar	45 mL
3 tbsp	frozen orange juice concentrate, thawed	45 mL
3 tbsp	olive oil	45 mL
2 tbsp	lemon juice	25 mL
2 tbsp	water	25 mL
1 ½ tsp	crushed garlic	7 mL
½ cup	chopped parsley	125 mL

1. Cook pasta in boiling water according to package instructions or until firm to the bite. Rinse with cold water. Drain and place in serving bowl.

2. Add sweet peppers, apricots, dates and green onions.

3. Make the dressing: In small bowl combine vinegar, orange juice concentrate, oil, lemon juice, water, garlic and parsley. Pour over salad, and toss.

MAKE AHEAD ◆ Prepare salad and dressing early in day. Toss just before serving.

If basil is unavailable, try spinach or parsley leaves.

◆

Roasted corn kernels (1 cob) make a delicious replacement for canned kernels. Broil or barbecue corn for 15 minutes or until charred.

Pesto Potato Salad

2 lb	scrubbed whole red potatoes with skins on	1 kg
PESTO		
1¼ cups	packed fresh basil leaves	300 mL
3 tbsp	olive oil	45 mL
2 tbsp	toasted pine nuts	25 mL
2 tbsp	grated Parmesan cheese	25 mL
1 tsp	minced garlic	5 mL
¼ tsp	salt	1 mL
¼ cup	chicken stock or water	50 mL
1 cup	halved snow peas	250 mL
¾ cup	chopped red onions	175 mL
¾ cup	chopped red peppers	175 mL
¾ cup	chopped green peppers	175 mL
½ cup	corn kernels	125 mL
2	medium green onions, chopped	2
2 tbsp	toasted pine nuts	25 mL
2 tbsp	lemon juice	25 mL

1. Put potatoes in saucepan with cold water to cover; bring to a boil and cook for 20 to 25 minutes, or until easily pierced with a sharp knife. Drain and set aside.

2. Meanwhile, put basil, olive oil, 2 tbsp (25 mL) pine nuts, Parmesan, garlic and salt in food processor; process until finely chopped. With the processor running, gradually add stock through the feed tube; process until smooth.

continued on page 71

3. In saucepan of boiling water or microwave, blanch snow peas for 1 or 2 minutes, or until tender-crisp; refresh in cold water and drain. Place in large serving bowl, along with pesto, red onions, red and green peppers, corn, green onions, 2 tbsp (25 mL) pine nuts and lemon juice. When potatoes are cool enough to handle, cut into wedges and add to serving bowl; toss well to combine.

MAKE AHEAD ◆ Prepare potatoes, pesto and vegetables up to a day ahead. Toss before serving. Tastes great the next day.

Mango Salsa over Vermicelli

8 oz	vermicelli or other fine-strand pasta	250 g
1¾ cups	diced mangoes	425 mL
¾ cup	diced sweet red peppers	175 mL
½ cup	diced red onions	125 mL
½ cup	diced sweet green peppers	125 mL
3 tbsp	olive oil	45 mL
3 tbsp	lemon juice	45 mL
2 tsp	crushed garlic	10 mL
½ cup	chopped coriander or parsley	125 mL

1. Cook pasta in boiling water according to package instructions or until firm to the bite. Rinse with cold water. Drain and set aside.

2. In bowl of food processor, combine mangoes, red peppers, onions, green peppers, oil, lemon juice, garlic and coriander. Process on and off just until finely diced. Pour over pasta; serve at room temperature.

MAKE AHEAD ◆ Prepare salsa early in day and refrigerate. (This will also allow it to develop more flavor.) Pour over pasta just before serving.

Split peas and rice are a dynamic combination.

◆

A nutrient filled main dish salad, this is an excellent source of magnesium, phosphorus, zinc, vitamins A and C, thiamin and folate and a good source of iron, riboflavin, niacin and pantothenic acid.

Split-Pea and Rice Greek Salad

4½ cups	basic vegetable stock (see recipe, page 46)	1.125 L
1 cup	dried green split peas	250 mL
1 cup	white or brown rice	250 mL
1½ cups	chopped tomatoes	375 mL
1 cup	chopped unpeeled cucumbers	250 mL
1 cup	chopped red bell peppers	250 mL
¾ cup	chopped red onions	175 mL
⅓ cup	sliced black olives	75 mL
3 oz	feta cheese, crumbled	75 g

DRESSING

2 tbsp	freshly squeezed lemon juice	25 mL
1½ tbsp	olive oil	20 mL
1 tbsp	balsamic vinegar	15 mL
1½ tsp	minced garlic	7 mL
1½ tsp	dried oregano	7 mL
½ tsp	coarsely ground black pepper	2 mL

1. In a saucepan bring 3 cups (750 mL) of the stock to a boil. Stir in split peas; reduce heat to medium and cook, covered, 25 to 35 minutes or until tender. Rinse under cold water and drain; set aside to cool.

2. Meanwhile, in a saucepan bring remaining 1½ cups (375 mL) stock to a boil. Stir in rice; reduce heat to low, cover and cook 20 minutes or until rice is tender and stock absorbed. (Brown rice will need 35 minutes and a little more stock.) Set aside to cool.

3. In a large serving bowl, combine tomatoes, cucumbers, red peppers, onions, olives, feta and cooled rice and split peas.

4. Make the dressing: In a small bowl, whisk together lemon juice, olive oil, balsamic vinegar, garlic, oregano and pepper. Pour over salad; toss to coat.

MAKE AHEAD ◆ Prepare early in the day.

PER SERVING

2½ ■ Starch Choices

1½ ◢ Fruit & Vegetable Choices

1 ◢ Protein Choice

1 ▲ Fat & Oil Choice

Calories 351
Carbohydrates . . . . 57 g
Fiber . . . . 6 g
Protein . . . . 14 g
Fat, total . . . . 9 g
Fat, saturated . . . . 3 g
Sodium . . . . 246 mg
Cholesterol . . . . . 13 mg

Fish and Seafood

Fish and seafood are excellent low-fat Protein choices. Research has shown that eating fish on a regular basis can be protective against cardiovascular disease. Fatty fish such as salmon and halibut are a good source of essential fatty acids.

What about seafood and cholesterol?

Many people have expressed concern about the cholesterol content of shrimp, lobster, crab and other seafood. While some of these do contain cholesterol, we need to be more concerned about the intake of saturated fat in the diet. This means eating less processed meat.

My recommendation to people with diabetes is to choose fish and seafood regularly as they are delicious and low in fat.

❖

Preheat oven to 425°F (220°C)

Baking sheet sprayed with nonstick vegetable spray

When making the pesto, use only parsley or only coriander leaves for an unusual taste.

◆

Salmon is a good source of Omega-3 fatty acids. Eating fatty fish high in Omega-3's is recommended weekly.

◆

This nutrient packed recipe provides an excellent source of Vitamin D, phosphorus, and the B vitamins; niacin, vitamin B_6 and B_{12}. It is also a good source of magnesium, vitamin C and pantothenic acid.

PER SERVING

4	⊘	Protein Choices
½	▲	Fat & Oil Choice

Calories 231
Carbohydrates . . . . . 1 g
Fiber . . . . 0 g
Protein . . . . 26 g
Fat, total . . . . 14 g
Fat, saturated . . . . 3 g
Sodium . . . . 103 mg
Cholesterol . . . . . 67 mg

Salmon with Pesto

1 lb	salmon steaks or fillet, cut into 4 serving-sized portions	500 g
1 tsp	vegetable oil	5 mL
1 tsp	lemon juice	5 mL
1 tsp	crushed garlic	5 mL
¼ cup	Pesto Sauce (recipe, page 163)	50 mL

1. Place salmon on baking sheet; brush with oil, lemon juice and garlic. Bake approximately 10 minutes or just until fish flakes easily when tested with fork.

2. Top each serving with 1 tbsp (15 mL) Pesto Sauce.

TIPS

Other white fish, such as sole, flounder or turbot, can be substituted.

◆

If using a thin piece of fish, you can probably skip the baking time. The fish will cook through in the skillet.

◆

Toast pecans either in 400°F (200°C) oven or in skillet on top of stove for 2 minutes or until brown.

Halibut with Lemon and Pecans

½ cup	bread crumbs	125 mL
1 tsp	dried parsley	5 mL
½ tsp	dried basil	2 mL
½ tsp	crushed garlic	2 mL
1½ tsp	grated Parmesan cheese	7 mL
1 lb	halibut, cut into 4 serving-sized pieces	500 g
1	egg white	1
2 tbsp	margarine	25 mL
2 tbsp	white wine	25 mL
4 tsp	lemon juice	20 mL
1 tbsp	chopped fresh parsley	15 mL
1	green onion, chopped	1
1 tbsp	chopped pecans, toasted	15 mL

1. In shallow dish, combine bread crumbs, dried parsley, basil, garlic and cheese. Dip fish pieces into egg white, then into bread crumb mixture.

2. In large nonstick skillet, melt 1 tbsp (15 mL) of the margarine; add fish and cook just until browned on both sides. Transfer fish to baking dish and bake for 5 to 10 minutes or until fish flakes easily when tested with fork. Remove to serving platter and keep warm.

3. To skillet, add remaining margarine, wine, lemon juice, parsley, onions and pecans; cook for 1 minute. Pour over fish.

PER SERVING

1	■ Starch Choice
4	◙ Protein Choices

Calories	275
Carbohydrates	13 g
Fiber	1 g
Protein	29 g
Fat, total	11 g
Fat, saturated	2 g
Sodium	274 mg
Cholesterol	41 mg

Red Snapper
with Broccoli and Dill Cheese Sauce

2 cups	chopped broccoli florets	500 mL
I lb	red snapper (or any firm fish fillets)	500 g
I tbsp	margarine	15 mL
I tbsp	all-purpose flour	15 mL
I cup	2% milk	250 mL
⅓ cup	shredded Cheddar cheese	75 mL
2 tbsp	chopped fresh dill (or ½ tsp [2 mL] dried dillweed)	25 mL
	Salt and pepper	

1. In boiling water, blanch broccoli until still crisp and color brightens; drain and place in baking dish. Place fish in single layer over top.

2. In small saucepan, melt margarine; add flour and cook, stirring, for 1 minute. Add milk and cook, stirring constantly, until thickened, approximately 3 minutes. Stir in cheese, dill, and salt and pepper to taste until cheese has melted; pour over fish.

3. Bake, uncovered, for 15 to 20 minutes or until fish flakes easily when tested with fork.

PER SERVING

½ ● Fruit & Vegetable Choice

I ◆ 2% Milk Choice

4½ ● Protein Choices

½ ▲ Fat & Oil Choice

Calories 306
Carbohydrates . . . . . 7 g
Fiber . . . . I g
Protein . . . . 34 g
Fat, total . . . . 15 g
Fat, saturated . . . . 6 g
Sodium . . . . 303 mg
Cholesterol . . . . 100 mg

Serves 4

Preheat oven to 425°F (220°C)

Baking dish sprayed with nonstick vegetable spray

TIPS

This tasty recipe is higher in carbohydrate than most fish dishes. A granulated sugar substitute can replace the brown sugar to eliminate the ½ ✱ Sugar choice or reduce the carbohydrate by about 5 g/serving.

◆

Any white fish is suitable. Try grouper, cod, halibut or haddock.

PER SERVING

2½ 🍃 Fruit & Vegetable Choices

½ ✱ Sugar Choice

3 🍖 Protein Choices

Calories 298
Carbohydrates . . . . 33 g
Fiber . . . . 2 g
Protein . . . . 23 g
Fat, total . . . . 12 g
Fat, saturated . . . . 1 g
Sodium . . . . 98 mg
Cholesterol . . . . . 42 mg

Fish Fillets with Apples, Raisins and Pecans

1 lb	firm white fish fillets	500 g
1 tbsp	margarine	15 mL
1 cup	chopped peeled apples	250 mL
⅓ cup	raisins	75 mL
¼ cup	chopped pecans or walnuts	50 mL
4 tsp	brown sugar	20 mL
½ tsp	cinnamon	2 mL
1 tbsp	all-purpose flour	15 mL
1 cup	apple juice	250 mL

1. Place fish in single layer in baking dish.

2. In nonstick skillet, melt margarine; sauté apples, raisins, pecans, sugar and cinnamon for 3 minutes or until apples are tender.

3. Mix flour with apple juice until dissolved; add to pan and cook until thickened, stirring constantly, 2 to 3 minutes.

4. Pour sauce over fish; cover and bake for approximately 15 minutes or until fish flakes easily when tested with fork.

Preheat oven to 400°F (200°C)

8-inch (2 L) square baking dish sprayed with vegetable spray

Salmon, trout or whitefish is ideal. Ask to have fish butterflied, scaled and deboned.

♦

At 6 ◙ Protein choices, this recipe may be more than the regular amount of protein you would choose at meal time. To compensate you may choose to reduce protein servings at another meal to maintain the same total energy intake.

PER SERVING

1½ ■ Starch Choices

1 ◢ Fruit & Vegetable Choice

½ ✳ Sugar Choice

6 ◙ Protein Choices

Calories 471

Carbohydrates . . . . 40 g

Fiber . . . . 2 g

Protein . . . . 45 g

Fat, total . . . . 13 g

Fat, saturated . . . . 2 g

Sodium . . . . 249 mg

Cholesterol . . . . 104 mg

Fish with Cornbread and Dill Stuffing

CORNBREAD

½ cup	cornmeal	125 mL
½ cup	all-purpose flour	125 mL
1½ tbsp	granulated sugar	20 mL
1½ tsp	baking powder	7 mL
¾ cup	2% yogurt	175 mL
¾ cup	corn kernels	175 mL
1	egg	1
1½ tbsp	melted margarine or butter	20 mL
2 tsp	vegetable oil	10 mL
1½ tsp	minced garlic	7 mL
1 cup	chopped onions	250 mL
1 cup	sliced mushrooms	250 mL
1 cup	chopped green or red peppers	250 mL
¼ cup	chopped fresh dill (or 2 tsp [10 mL] dried)	50 mL
1	whole 2-lb (1 kg) fish, rinsed under cold water	1
1 tsp	vegetable oil	5 mL
1 tsp	minced garlic	5 mL
⅓ cup	chicken stock or water	75 mL
⅓ cup	white wine	75 mL

1. In large bowl stir together cornmeal, flour, sugar and baking powder. In another bowl combine yogurt, corn, egg and margarine. Add the wet ingredients to the dry ingredients and stir just until combined. Pour batter into prepared pan and bake for 15 to 18 minutes or until cake tester inserted in center comes out clean.

2. In nonstick skillet sprayed with vegetable spray, heat oil over medium heat. Add garlic and onion and cook for 4 minutes or until softened. Add mushrooms and peppers and cook for 5 minutes or until vegetables are tender. Stir in dill and remove from heat.

continued on page 79

3. Crumble the cooled cornbread into a large bowl. Add vegetable mixture and combine thoroughly. Stuff half of the mixture into fish. Place remaining mixture in dish and serve warmed with fish. Place fish in baking pan sprayed with vegetable spray and brush fish with oil and garlic. Pour stock and wine into pan. Cover and bake for 35 to 45 minutes or until fish flakes easily when pierced with a fork.

MAKE AHEAD ◆ Prepare entire stuffing with vegetables up to one day in advance.

Serves 6

Start barbecue or preheat oven to 425°F (220°C)

Swordfish with Mango Coriander Salsa

1 ½ lbs	swordfish steaks	750 g
1 tsp	vegetable oil	5 mL
SALSA		
1 ½ cups	finely diced mango or peach	375 mL
¾ cup	finely diced red peppers	175 mL
½ cup	finely diced green peppers	125 mL
½ cup	finely diced red onions	125 mL
¼ cup	chopped fresh coriander	50 mL
2 tbsp	lemon juice	25 mL
2 tsp	olive oil	10 mL
1 tsp	minced garlic	5 mL

1. Brush fish with 1 tsp (5 mL) of oil on both sides. Barbecue or bake fish for 10 minutes per inch (2.5 cm) thickness, or until it flakes easily when pierced with a fork.

2. Meanwhile, in bowl combine mango, red peppers, green peppers, red onions, coriander, lemon juice, olive oil and garlic; mix thoroughly. Serve over fish.

MAKE AHEAD ◆ Make salsa early in the day and refrigerate.

PER SERVING

1	🍎 Fruit & Vegetable Choice
3½	🍖 Protein Choices

Calories	219
Carbohydrates	12 g
Fiber	2 g
Protein	26 g
Fat, total	8 g
Fat, saturated	2 g
Sodium	111 mg
Cholesterol	49 mg

Try to make the relish as close to the time of serving as possible; otherwise the cucumber will make the sauce too watery.

◆

Use cod, snapper or haddock.

◆

Use 1 ½ tsp (7 mL) dried dill if fresh is unavailable.

◆

The flatter the fish, the faster it cooks.

Crunchy Fish
with Cucumber Dill Relish

RELISH

2 cups	finely chopped cucumbers	500 mL
1/3 cup	chopped fresh dill	75 mL
1/3 cup	2% yogurt	75 mL
1/4 cup	finely diced green onions (about 2 medium)	50 mL
1/4 cup	finely diced green peppers	50 mL
3 tbsp	light mayonnaise	45 mL
I tsp	minced garlic	5 mL

CRUNCHY FISH

2 cups	corn flakes	500 mL
I tbsp	grated Parmesan cheese	15 mL
I tsp	minced garlic	5 mL
1/2 tsp	dried basil	2 mL
I	egg	I
3 tbsp	2% milk	45 mL
3 tbsp	all-purpose flour	45 mL
I lb	firm white fish fillets	500 g
I tbsp	margarine or butter	15 mL

1. Relish: In bowl, combine cucumbers, dill, yogurt, green onions, green peppers, mayonnaise and garlic; mix to combine and set aside.

2. Put corn flakes, Parmesan, garlic and basil in food processor; process until fine and put on a plate. In shallow bowl whisk together egg and milk. Dust fish with flour.

3. Dip fish fillets in egg wash, then coat with crumb mixture. In large nonstick skillet sprayed with vegetable spray, melt margarine over medium heat. Add fillets and cook for 5 minutes or until browned, turn and cook for 2 minutes longer, or until fish is browned and flakes easily when pierced with a fork. Serve topped with cucumber dill relish.

MAKE AHEAD ◆ Prepare fish early in the day and keep refrigerated until ready to bake.

The shells of mussels should be tightly closed when buying.

◆

Fresh juicy tomatoes are excellent when in season.

◆

Substitute clams for the mussels.

◆

An excellent source of vitamin B$_{12}$, this recipe also is a good source of iron and vitamin C. The body will absorb more iron when vitamin C is present.

Mussels with Tomatoes, Basil and Garlic

2 lb	mussels	1 kg
1 ½ tsp	vegetable oil	7 mL
½ cup	finely diced onions	125 mL
2 tsp	crushed garlic	10 mL
1	can (14 oz [398 mL]) tomatoes, drained and chopped	1
⅓ cup	dry white wine	75 mL
1 tbsp	chopped fresh basil (or ½ tsp [2 mL] dried)	15 mL
1 ½ tsp	chopped fresh oregano (or ¼ tsp [1 mL] dried)	7 mL

1. Scrub mussels under cold water; pull off hairy beards. Discard any that do not close when tapped. Set aside.

2. In large nonstick saucepan, heat oil; sauté onions and garlic for 2 minutes. Add tomatoes, wine, basil and oregano; cook for 3 minutes, stirring constantly.

3. Add mussels; cover and cook until mussels fully open, 4 to 5 minutes. Discard any that do not open. Arrange mussels in bowls; pour sauce over top.

PER SERVING

| 1 | Fruit & Vegetable Choice |
| 1 | Protein Choice |

Calories 117
Carbohydrates . . . . 12 g
Fiber . . . . 2 g
Protein . . . . 8 g
Fat, total . . . . 3 g
Fat, saturated . . . . 0 g
Sodium . . . . 421 mg
Cholesterol . . . . . 15 mg

Imitation crab is less expensive than real crab meat. However, real crab (or cooked, chopped shrimp) can also be used. This dish can be served as an appetizer or as an entrée.

◆

Both the imitation crab and seasoned dried bread crumbs are significant sources of sodium in this recipe. You can reduce this by using plain dry bread crumbs.

PER SERVING

1	■ Starch Choice	
½	◖ Fruit & Vegetable Choice	
3	◉ Protein Choices	
½	▲ Fat & Oil Choice	

Calories 272
Carbohydrates . . . . 20 g
Fiber . . . . 1 g
Protein . . . . 22 g
Fat, total . . . . 11 g
Fat, saturated . . . . 2 g
Sodium . . . . 1336 mg
Cholesterol . . . . . 98 mg

Sautéed Crab Cakes
with Chunky Dill Tartar Sauce

½ tsp	vegetable oil	2 tsp
1 tsp	minced garlic	5 mL
½ cup	chopped onions	125 mL
12 oz	imitation crab (sea legs, Krab legs or Krab flakes)	375 g
⅔ cup	seasoned bread crumbs	150 mL
¼ cup	chopped fresh dill (or 2 tsp [10 mL] dried)	50 mL
1	whole egg	1
1	egg white	1
2 tbsp	light mayonnaise	25 mL
2 tsp	lemon juice	10 mL
1 tbsp	margarine or butter	15 mL

CHUNKY DILL TARTAR SAUCE

3 tbsp	light mayonnaise	45 mL
3 tbsp	light sour cream	45 mL
2 tbsp	finely chopped green peppers	25 mL
2 tbsp	finely chopped red onions	25 mL
2 tbsp	chopped fresh dill (or ½ tsp [2 mL] dried)	25 mL
2 tsp	lemon juice	10 mL

1. Heat oil in small nonstick skillet over medium heat; add garlic and onions and cook for 5 minutes or until softened. Put in food processor along with crab, bread crumbs, dill, whole egg, egg white, mayonnaise and lemon juice. Pulse on and off until finely chopped. Form each ⅓ cup (75 mL) into a patty.

2. Sauce: In small bowl combine mayonnaise, sour cream, green peppers, onions, dill and lemon juice; set aside.

continued on page 83

3. Melt margarine in large nonstick skillet sprayed with vegetable spray over medium heat. Add crab cakes and cook for 6 minutes, or until golden; turn and cook for 6 minutes longer, or until golden and hot. Serve with chunky dill tartar sauce.

MAKE AHEAD ◆ Prepare crab mixture and sauce earlier in the day. They can also be cooked in advance and gently reheated.

Scallops with Basil Tomato Sauce

1 tbsp	margarine	15 mL
¾ cup	chopped onions	175 mL
1 tsp	crushed garlic	5 mL
¾ cup	diced sweet green pepper	175 mL
¾ cup	sliced mushrooms	175 mL
2 tsp	all-purpose flour	10 mL
1 cup	2% milk	250 mL
2 tbsp	tomato paste	25 mL
1¼ tsp	dried basil (or 2 tbsp [25 mL] chopped fresh)	6 mL
1 lb	scallops, sliced in half if large	500 g
1 tbsp	grated Parmesan cheese	15 mL

1. In large nonstick skillet, melt margarine; sauté onions, garlic, green pepper and mushrooms until softened, approximately 5 minutes. Stir in flour and cook for 1 minute, stirring.

2. Add milk, tomato paste and basil; cook, stirring continuously, until thickened, 2 to 3 minutes.

3. Add scallops; cook just until opaque, 2 to 3 minutes. Place on serving dish; sprinkle with Parmesan cheese.

Serves 6

Preheat oven to 350°F (180°C)

10- to 11-inch (3L) springform pan sprayed with vegetable spray

PER SERVING

1½ ▪ Starch Choices

½ ▰ Fruit & Vegetable Choice

3 ▣ Protein Choices

½ ▲ Fat & Oil Choice

Calories 309
Carbohydrates . . . . 28 g
Fiber . . . . 1 g
Protein . . . . 24 g
Fat, total . . . . 11 g
Fat, saturated . . . . 6 g
Sodium . . . . 521 mg
Cholesterol . . . . 123 mg

Seafood Pasta Pizza
with Dill and Goat Cheese

6 oz	broken linguine	150 g
1	egg	1
⅓ cup	2% milk	75 mL
3 tbsp	grated Parmesan cheese	45 mL
8 oz	seafood, cut in pieces or left whole (shrimp, scallops, squid)	250 g
1 tsp	vegetable oil	5 mL
1½ tsp	crushed garlic	7 mL
¾ cup	diced sweet red peppers	175 mL
¼ cup	chopped green onions	50 mL
¼ cup	sliced red onions	50 mL
1 cup	cold seafood or chicken stock	250 mL
1 cup	2% milk	250 mL
3 tbsp	all-purpose flour	45 mL
⅓ cup	chopped fresh dill (or 1 tbsp [15 mL] dried)	75 mL
½ cup	shredded mozzarella cheese	125 mL
2 oz	goat cheese, crumbled	50 g

1. Cook pasta in boiling water according to package instructions or until firm to the bite. Drain and place in mixing bowl. Add egg, milk and cheese. Mix well. Pour into pan and bake for 20 minutes.

2. In large nonstick skillet sprayed with vegetable spray, sauté seafood just until cooked, approximately 3 minutes. Drain and set seafood aside.

3. In same skillet, heat oil; sauté garlic, red peppers and green and red onions for 4 minutes.

continued on page 85

4. Meanwhile, in small bowl combine stock, milk and flour until smooth. Add to skillet and simmer on low heat until thickened, approximately 2 minutes, stirring constantly. Add dill and seafood. Pour into pan. Sprinkle with mozzarella and goat cheese; bake for 10 minutes. Let rest for 10 minutes before serving.

MAKE AHEAD ◆ Crust can be made a day ahead and covered. Filling can be made ahead; add more stock if too thick.

There are many combinations of seafood which can be used. A more economical version can be made by combining a firm white fish such as cod, grouper or halibut with some of the seafood.

◆

Freeze shrimp with their shells to preserve the best taste.

PER SERVING		
½ ⬛ Fruit & Vegetable Choice		
4 ⬛ Protein Choices		
Calories 260		
Carbohydrates . . . . . 5 g		
Fiber . . . . 0 g		
Protein . . . . 30 g		
Fat, total . . . . 12 g		
Fat, saturated . . . . 4 g		
Sodium . . . . 316 mg		
Cholesterol . . . . 199 mg		

Shrimp and Scallops
with Cheesy Cream Sauce

1 tbsp	margarine	15 mL
1 tsp	crushed garlic	5 mL
⅓ cup	chopped green onions	75 mL
1 lb	seafood (shrimp, scallops or combination)	500 g
¼ cup	chopped fresh parsley	50 mL
2 oz	goat or feta cheese, crumbled	50 g
SAUCE		
1 tbsp	margarine	15 mL
2½ tsp	all-purpose flour	12 mL
⅓ cup	dry white wine	75 mL
½ cup	2% milk	125 mL

1. Sauce: In small saucepan, melt margarine; stir in flour and cook, stirring, for 1 minute. Add wine and milk; cook, stirring, until thickened and smooth, approximately 2 minutes. Set aside and keep warm.

2. In nonstick skillet, melt margarine; sauté garlic, green onions and seafood just until seafood is opaque. Remove from stove; add sauce and mix well.

3. Pour into serving dish; sprinkle parsley and cheese over top.

Replace squid with shrimp, scallops or lobster.

◆

For a spicier version, add ¼ tsp (1 mL) cayenne pepper.

◆

Complete the meal with a salad composed of ❖❖ Extra Vegetables and low-fat dressing.

Pasta with Squid and Clams in a Spicy Tomato Sauce

12 oz	spaghetti	375 g
2 tsp	vegetable oil	10 mL
1½ tsp	crushed garlic	7 mL
1 cup	chopped onions	250 mL
1 cup	chopped sweet green peppers	250 mL
1	can (19 oz [540 mL]) crushed tomatoes	1
2	cans (5 oz [142 mL]) baby clams, liquid reserved from 1 can	2
1 tbsp	tomato paste	15 mL
2 tsp	capers	10 mL
1½ tsp	dried basil	7 mL
¾ tsp	dried oregano	4 mL
2 tsp	chili powder	10 mL
12 oz	squid, cleaned and sliced	375 g
3 tbsp	grated Parmesan cheese Parsley	45 mL

1. Cook pasta in boiling water according to package instructions or until firm to the bite. Drain and place in serving bowl.

2. In large nonstick saucepan, heat oil; sauté garlic, onions and green peppers until soft, approximately 5 minutes. Add crushed tomatoes, liquid from 1 can of clams, tomato paste, capers, basil, oregano and chili powder. Cover and simmer on low heat until thick, for 15 to 20 minutes, stirring occasionally. Add clams and squid; simmer just until squid is cooked, approximately 3 minutes. Pour over pasta. Sprinkle with cheese, and toss. Garnish with parsley.

MAKE AHEAD ◆ Prepare sauce a day ahead up to point where seafood is added. Reheat gently, then continue with recipe.

PER SERVING

3 ▣ Starch Choices

1½ ◪ Fruit & Vegetable Choices

3½ ◪ Protein Choices

Calories 445
Carbohydrates . . . . 65 g
Fiber . . . . 4 g
Protein . . . . 33 g
Fat, total . . . . 6 g
Fat, saturated . . . . 1 g
Sodium . . . . 439 mg
Cholesterol . . . . 180 mg

Shrimp can be replaced with scallops, squid or firm fish fillets such as orange roughy or halibut.

◆

Chicken can be substituted for fish.

◆

Goat cheese can replace feta cheese. Walnuts, pecans or cashews can replace pine nuts.

Linguine with Shrimp, Red Peppers and Pine Nuts

8 oz	linguine	250 g
8 oz	shrimp, shelled, deveined and cut into pieces	250 g
2 tsp	vegetable oil	10 mL
2 tsp	crushed garlic	10 mL
2 cups	chopped sweet red peppers	500 mL
1/3 cup	chopped green onions	75 mL
1/2 cup	chopped fresh basil (or 2 tsp [10 mL] dried)	125 mL
1 1/2 tsp	dried oregano	7 mL
1 1/4 cups	cold fish or chicken stock	300 mL
3 1/2 tsp	all-purpose flour	17 mL
3 1/2 oz	feta cheese, crumbled	90 g
2 tbsp	toasted pine nuts	25 mL

1. Cook pasta in boiling water according to package instructions or until firm to the bite. Drain and place in serving bowl.

2. In medium nonstick skillet sprayed with nonstick vegetable spray, sauté shrimp just until pink and just cooked, approximately 3 minutes. Drain and add to pasta.

3. In large nonstick skillet, heat oil; sauté garlic and red peppers for 3 minutes. Add onions, basil and oregano; sauté for 3 minutes.

4. Meanwhile, in small bowl, combine stock and flour until smooth. Add to red pepper mixture; simmer, stirring constantly until thickened, approximately 3 minutes. Add cheese and allow to melt. Pour over pasta. Add pine nuts, and toss.

MAKE AHEAD ◆ Prepare sauce in Steps 3 and 4 early in day. Do not add cheese. Reheat gently. Add cheese and continue with recipe.

PER SERVING

3 ■ Starch Choices

1 ◢ Fruit & Vegetable Choice

2 1/2 ◉ Protein Choices

1/2 ▲ Fat & Oil Choice

Calories 430
Carbohydrates . . . . 57 g
Fiber . . . . 3 g
Protein . . . . 26 g
Fat, total . . . . 11 g
Fat, saturated . . . . 5 g
Sodium . . . . 807 mg
Cholesterol . . . . 118 mg

The shrimp can be replaced with scallops or a combination of both.

◆

This delicious recipe is chock full of nutrients too. It is an excellent source of magnesium, phosphorus, iron, vitamins A, niacin, B_{12} and C and a good source of zinc, vitamin B_6 and folic acid.

Chinese Shrimp Sauté
with Green Onions and Pecans

1 ½ cups	chopped broccoli florets	375 mL
1 ½ cups	snow peas, trimmed	375 mL
⅔ cup	chicken stock	150 mL
2 tbsp	hoisin sauce	25 mL
1 tbsp	cornstarch	15 mL
1 tsp	minced gingerroot (or ½ tsp [2 mL] ground)	5 mL
1 tbsp	olive oil	15 mL
1 ½ tsp	crushed garlic	7 mL
¾ cup	chopped sweet red pepper	175 mL
1 lb	medium shrimp, peeled and deveined	500 g
1 tbsp	chopped pecans	15 mL
1	green onion, finely chopped	1

1. Blanch broccoli and snow peas in boiling water just until color brightens; drain and set aside.

2. Combine chicken stock, hoisin sauce, cornstarch and ginger until mixed. Set aside.

3. In large skillet, heat oil; sauté garlic and red pepper for 2 minutes. Add shrimp and hoisin mixture; sauté just until shrimp turns pink and sauce thickens. Add broccoli, snow peas and pecans; toss well. Sprinkle with green onions.

PER SERVING

1	▣	Fruit & Vegetable Choice
4	▣	Protein Choices
1	✦✦	Extra Choice

Calories 245
Carbohydrates . . . . 15 g
Fiber . . . . 3 g
Protein . . . . 29 g
Fat, total . . . . 8 g
Fat, saturated . . . . 1 g
Sodium . . . . 535 mg
Cholesterol . . . . 190 mg

Poultry

Chicken is a lean meat that goes well with a variety of vegetables and tastes. A good source of low-fat Protein choices, the majority of recipes begin with boneless skinless chicken breasts. In fact one (3 oz/100 g) boneless skinless chicken breast roasted contains only 2.1 g of fat (or less than ½ teaspoon) and is a source of more than 10 vitamins and minerals. The mouth-watering recipes which follow provide some new alternatives to "traditional" chicken meals and are sure to become some of your family favorites.

❖

Preheat oven to 375°F
(190°C)

Baking dish sprayed
with nonstick
vegetable spray

Try yellow pepper
instead of the red.

◆

Fresh herbs will last
longer if placed in a glass
with some water
covering the stems and
plastic wrap to cover
the glass. Store in
the refrigerator.

PER SERVING

½ ▣ Starch Choices

1½ ▰ Fruit & Vegetable
Choices

3 ▰ Protein Choices

Calories 193
Carbohydrates . . . . . 8 g
Fiber . . . . 1 g
Protein . . . . 21 g
Fat, total . . . . 8 g
Fat, saturated . . . . 2 g
Sodium . . . . 266 mg
Cholesterol . . . . . 51 mg

Chicken Breasts
Stuffed with Red Pepper Purée in Creamy Sauce

4	boneless skinless chicken breasts	4
1 tbsp	vegetable oil	15 mL
½ tsp	crushed garlic	2 mL
¾ cup	diced sweet red pepper	175 mL
1 tbsp	water	15 mL
2 tbsp	chopped fresh dill (or ½ tsp [2 mL] dried dillweed)	25 mL
2 tbsp	dry bread crumbs	25 mL
1½ tsp	grated Parmesan cheese	7 mL
1 tbsp	toasted pine nuts	15 mL
	Salt and pepper	
¼ cup	chicken stock or water	50 mL
SAUCE		
1½ tsp	margarine	7 mL
1½ tsp	all-purpose flour	7 mL
¾ cup	2% milk	175 mL
1 tbsp	grated Parmesan cheese	15 mL
1 tbsp	chopped fresh dill (or ¼ tsp [1 mL] dried dillweed)	15 mL
Pinch	paprika	Pinch

1. Place chicken between 2 sheets of waxed paper; pound until flattened. Set aside.

2. In nonstick skillet, heat oil; sauté garlic and red pepper for 3 minutes; stir in water. Transfer to food processor and purée; pour into bowl. Stir in dill, bread crumbs, cheese, pine nuts, and salt and pepper to taste, mixing well and adding a little water if too dry.

3. Divide purée among chicken breasts; roll up and fasten with toothpicks. Place in baking dish; pour in stock. Cover and bake for about 15 minutes or until chicken is no longer pink inside. Transfer to serving dish.

continued on page 91

4. Sauce: Meanwhile, in saucepan, melt margarine; add flour and cook, stirring, for 1 minute. Gradually add milk and cook, stirring, until thickened, approximately 3 minutes. Stir in cheese, dill and paprika. Pour over chicken.

MAKE AHEAD ◆ Assemble stuffed breasts early in day and refrigerate. Bake just before serving. Prepare sauce early in day and reheat gently, adding a little more milk if too thick.

Serves 4

TIPS

This tart yet sweet marinade complements veal and firm white fish, too.

◆

For a change, try a combination of red or yellow pepper instead of the green pepper.

◆

Serve over a bed of brown rice.

PER SERVING

1	🍃 Fruit & Vegetable Choice	
½	✳ Sugar Choice	
1½	◉ Protein Choices	
½	▲ Fat & Oil Choice	

Calories 165
Carbohydrates . . . . 16 g
Fiber . . . . 2 g
Protein . . . . 11 g
Fat, total . . . . 7 g
Fat, saturated . . . . . . 1 g
Sodium . . . . 31 mg
Cholesterol . . . . . 26 mg

Chicken Kabobs
with Ginger Lemon Marinade

8 oz	boneless skinless chicken breasts, cut into 2-inch (5 cm) cubes	250 g
16	squares sweet green pepper	16
16	pineapple chunks (fresh or canned)	16
16	cherry tomatoes	16

GINGER LEMON MARINADE

3 tbsp	lemon juice	45 mL
2 tbsp	water	25 mL
1 tbsp	vegetable oil	15 mL
2 tsp	sesame oil	10 mL
1½ tsp	red wine vinegar	7 mL
4 tsp	brown sugar	20 mL
1 tsp	minced gingerroot (or ¼ tsp [1 mL] ground)	5 mL
½ tsp	ground coriander	2 mL
½ tsp	ground fennel seeds (optional)	2 mL

1. Ginger Lemon Marinade: In small bowl, combine lemon juice, water, vegetable oil, sesame oil, vinegar, brown sugar, ginger, coriander, and fennel seeds (if using); mix well. Add chicken and mix well; marinate for 20 minutes.

2. Alternately thread chicken cubes, green pepper, pineapple and tomatoes onto 4 long or 8 short barbecue skewers. Barbecue for 15 to 20 minutes or just until chicken is no longer pink inside, brushing often with marinade and rotating every 5 minutes.

Preheat oven to 425°F (220°C)

Baking dish sprayed with nonstick vegetable spray

Chicken quarters or breasts with the bone in can also be used. Bake for 20 to 30 minutes or until no longer pink inside.

◆

The 3 tbsp (45 mL) brown sugar in this recipe contribute 1 ✳ Sugar Choice to this recipe. Substituting a low-calorie sugar substitute can eliminate the Sugar choice from this recipe, altering the taste slightly.

PER SERVING

½ ▣ Fruit & Vegetable Choice

1 ✳ Sugar Choice

3 ▣ Protein Choices

Calories 243
Carbohydrates . . . . 17 g
Fiber . . . . 1 g
Protein . . . . 21 g
Fat, total . . . . 10 g
Fat, saturated . . . . 1 g
Sodium . . . . 536 mg
Cholesterol . . . . . 48 mg

Chicken with
Teriyaki Vegetables

4	boneless skinless chicken breasts	4
1 tsp	vegetable oil	5 mL
1 tsp	crushed garlic	5 mL
1	large sweet red pepper, sliced thinly	1
1 cup	snow peas, trimmed	250 mL

MARINADE

3 tbsp	sherry	45 mL
3 tbsp	brown sugar	45 mL
2 tbsp	water	25 mL
2 tbsp	soya sauce	25 mL
2 tbsp	vegetable oil	25 mL
1½ tsp	minced gingerroot	7 mL

1. Marinade: In medium bowl, combine sherry, sugar, water, soya sauce, oil and ginger. Set aside.

2. Place chicken between 2 sheets of waxed paper; pound until thin and flattened. Add to bowl and marinate for 30 minutes.

3. Remove chicken and place in baking dish. Pour marinade into saucepan; cook for 3 to 4 minutes or until thickened and syrupy. Set 2 tbsp (25 mL) aside; brush remainder over chicken. Cover and bake for 10 to 15 minutes or until no longer pink inside.

4. Meanwhile, in large nonstick skillet, heat oil; sauté garlic, red pepper and snow peas for 2 minutes. Add reserved marinade; cook for 2 minutes, stirring constantly. Serve over chicken.

Preheat oven to broil

Baking sheet sprayed with vegetable spray

Use 4 oz (125 g) of bottled roasted red peppers packed in water rather than roasting your own.

◆

Serve chicken breasts whole or slice crosswise into medallions and fan out on the plate for a pretty presentation.

◆

Reduce the sodium content of the recipe by substituting plain dry crumbs for the seasoned ones.

◆

If prosciutto is unavailable, use thin slices of smoked ham.

◆

If a more intense flavor is desired, use a stronger tasting cheese.

PER SERVING

1	■ Starch Choice	
4	◪ Protein Choices	
1	✚✚ Extra Choice	

Calories 258
Carbohydrates . . . . 17 g
Fiber . . . . 0 g
Protein . . . . 30 g
Fat, total . . . . 7 g
Fat, saturated . . . . 2 g
Sodium . . . . 714 mg
Cholesterol . . . . . 65 mg

Chicken with Roasted Pepper and Prosciutto

1	small red pepper	1
1 lb	skinless, boneless chicken breasts (about 4)	500 g
1 oz	sliced prosciutto (4 thin slices)	25 g
2 oz	mozzarella cheese, cut into 4 equal-sized pieces	50 g
1	egg white	1
2 tbsp	water	25 mL
⅔ cup	seasoned bread crumbs	150 mL
2 tsp	vegetable oil	10 mL

1. Broil red pepper for 15 to 20 minutes, turning often until charred on all sides. Preheat oven to 425°F (220°C). Put pepper in bowl and cover tightly with plastic wrap. When cool enough to handle, remove stem, skin and seeds, and cut into thin strips.

2. Pound chicken breasts between sheets of waxed paper to ¼-inch (5-mm) thickness. Divide prosciutto slices among flattened chicken breasts. Place a piece of cheese at the short end of each breast, and place roasted pepper strips on top of the cheese. Starting at the filling end, carefully roll the breasts up tightly. Use a toothpick to hold chicken breast together.

3. In small bowl, whisk together egg white and water. Put bread crumbs on a plate. Dip each chicken roll in egg white mixture, then in bread crumbs. Heat oil in nonstick skillet sprayed with vegetable spray. Cook over high heat for 3 minutes, turning often, or until browned on all sides. Transfer to prepared baking sheet and bake for 10 to 15 minutes. Remove toothpicks before serving.

MAKE AHEAD ◆ Assemble chicken breasts early in the day, and refrigerate before baking. Bake 5 minutes longer due to refrigeration.

Try other nuts, such as cashews or pecans.

♦

Try veal or turkey scallopini instead of chicken.

♦

Serve with couscous and Green Beans and Diced Tomatoes (page 146) for an eye-catching meal.

Almond Chicken Breasts with Creamy Tarragon Mustard Sauce

1 lb	skinless, boneless chicken breasts	500 g
3 tbsp	all-purpose flour	45 mL
1	egg white	1
3 tbsp	water	45 mL
1/3 cup	finely chopped almonds	75 mL
1/2 cup	seasoned bread crumbs	125 mL
2 tsp	vegetable oil	10 mL
SAUCE		
1/4 cup	light mayonnaise	50 mL
1/4 cup	light sour cream	50 mL
1 tsp	Dijon mustard	5 mL
1 tsp	dried tarragon	5 mL

1. Between sheets of waxed paper, pound breasts to 1/4-inch (5-mm) thickness. Dust with flour. In shallow bowl, whisk together egg white and water. Combine almonds and bread crumbs and place on a plate.

2. In nonstick skillet sprayed with vegetable spray, heat oil over medium-high heat. Dip breasts in egg wash, then in crumb mixture. Cook for 3 minutes on one side; turn and cook for 2 minutes longer or until just done at center.

3. Meanwhile, in small saucepan whisk together mayonnaise, sour cream, mustard and tarragon; heat over low heat just until warm. Serve over chicken.

MAKE AHEAD ♦ Bread chicken breasts and prepare sauce earlier in the day. Cook just before serving.

PER SERVING

1	■	Starch Choice
1/2	✳	Sugar Choice
3 1/2	◕	Protein Choices
1 1/2	▲	Fat & Oil Choices

Calories 340
Carbohydrates . . . . 19 g
Fiber . . . . 2 g
Protein . . . . 27 g
Fat, total . . . . 17 g
Fat, saturated . . . . 3 g
Sodium . . . . 536 mg
Cholesterol . . . . . 61 mg

Preheat oven to 425°F
(220°C)

Baking sheet sprayed
with vegetable spray

Turkey, veal or pork
scallopini can
replace chicken.

◆

A stronger cheese, such
as Swiss, can replace
mozzarella.

◆

A great dish to reheat
the next day.

◆

The chicken together
with the cheese in the
recipe provide 4½ 🔘
Protein choices. If your
meal plan calls for less,
use smaller chicken
breasts in the recipe.

PER SERVING

1	■	Starch Choice
½	🔘	Fruit & Vegetable Choice
4½	🔘	Protein Choices

Calories 325
Carbohydrates . . . . 19 g
Fiber . . . . 0 g
Protein . . . . 35 g
Fat, total . . . . 11 g
Fat, saturated . . . . 5 g
Sodium . . . . 924 mg
Cholesterol . . . . 127 mg

Chicken and Eggplant Parmesan

4	crosswise slices of eggplant, skin on, approximately ½ inch (1 cm) thick	4
1	whole egg	1
1	egg white	1
1 tbsp	water or milk	15 mL
⅔ cup	seasoned bread crumbs	150 mL
3 tbsp	chopped fresh parsley (or 2 tsp [10 mL] dried)	45 mL
1 tbsp	grated Parmesan cheese	15 mL
1 lb	skinless, boneless chicken breasts (about 4)	500 g
2 tsp	vegetable oil	10 mL
1 tsp	minced garlic	5 mL
½ cup	tomato pasta sauce	125 mL
½ cup	grated mozzarella cheese	125 mL

1. In small bowl, whisk together whole egg, egg white and water. On plate stir together bread crumbs, parsley and Parmesan. Dip eggplant slices in egg wash, then coat with bread-crumb mixture. Place on prepared pan and bake for 20 minutes, or until tender, turning once.

2. Meanwhile, pound chicken breasts between sheets of waxed paper to ¼-inch (5-mm) thickness. Dip chicken in remaining egg wash, then coat with remaining bread-crumb mixture. Heat oil and garlic in nonstick skillet sprayed with vegetable spray and cook for 4 minutes, or until golden brown, turning once.

3. Spread 1 tbsp (15 mL) of tomato sauce on each eggplant slice. Place one chicken breast on top of each eggplant slice. Spread another 1 tbsp (15 mL) of tomato sauce on top of each chicken piece. Sprinkle with cheese and bake for 5 minutes or until cheese melts.

MAKE AHEAD ◆ Prepare earlier in the day, refrigerate and bake at 350°F (180°C) until warm (approximately 10 minutes).

Preheat oven to 400°F
(200°C)

PER SERVING

2	■	Starch Choices
2	◪	Fruit & Vegetable Choices
2	◪	Protein Choices

Calories 362
Carbohydrates . . . . 55 g
Fiber . . . . 7 g
Protein . . . . 22 g
Fat, total . . . . 5 g
Fat, saturated . . . . 1 g
Sodium . . . . 591 mg
Cholesterol . . . . . 46 mg

Chicken with Leeks, Sweet Potatoes and Dates

4	chicken breasts or legs	4
	All-purpose flour for dusting	
1 tbsp	margarine	15 mL
2 tsp	crushed garlic	10 mL
2 cups	chopped leeks	500 mL
2 cups	chopped peeled sweet potatoes	500 mL
1½ cups	chicken stock	375 mL
⅓ cup	white wine	75 mL
½ tsp	cinnamon	2 mL
½ tsp	ground ginger	2 mL
½ cup	chopped dates	125 mL

1. Dust chicken with flour. In nonstick skillet sprayed with nonstick vegetable spray, brown chicken on both sides, approximately 10 minutes. Place in baking dish.

2. In same skillet, melt margarine; sauté garlic, leeks and potatoes until softened, approximately 10 minutes, stirring constantly. Add chicken stock, wine, cinnamon and ginger; cover and simmer for 10 minutes. Stir in dates.

3. Pour sauce over chicken; bake for 20 to 30 minutes, basting occasionally, or until chicken is no longer pink inside and juices run clear when chicken is pierced. Remove skin before eating.

Curried Lamb Casserole ➤
with Sweet Potatoes (page 116)
Overleaf: Rotini with Tomatoes,
Black Olives and Goat Cheese (page 121)

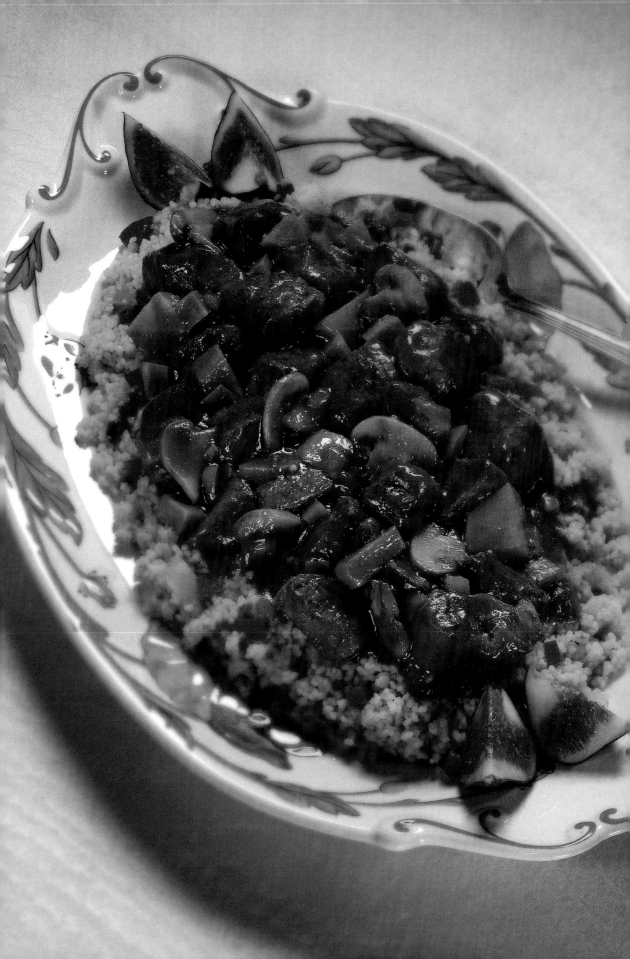

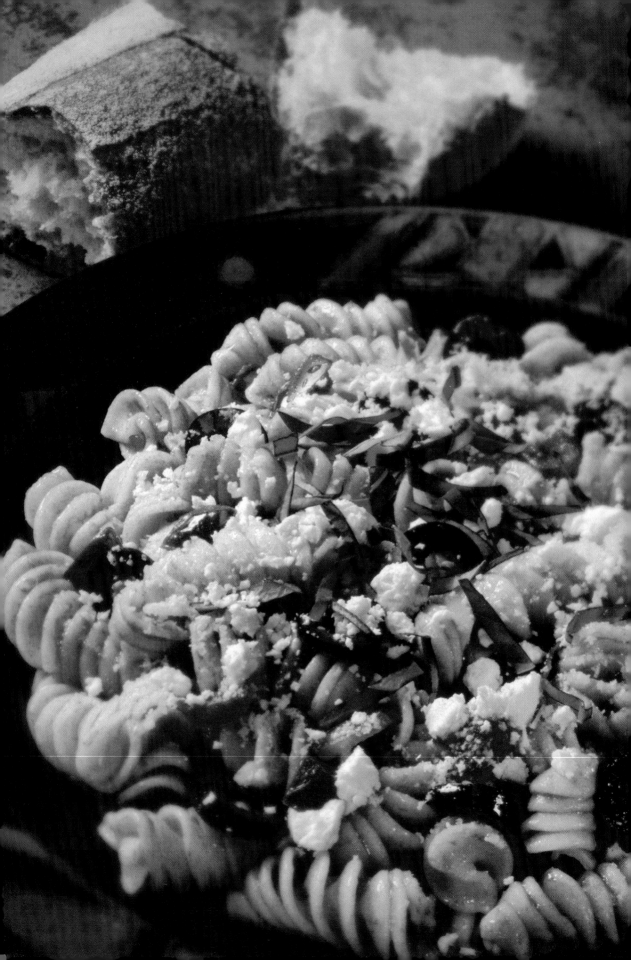

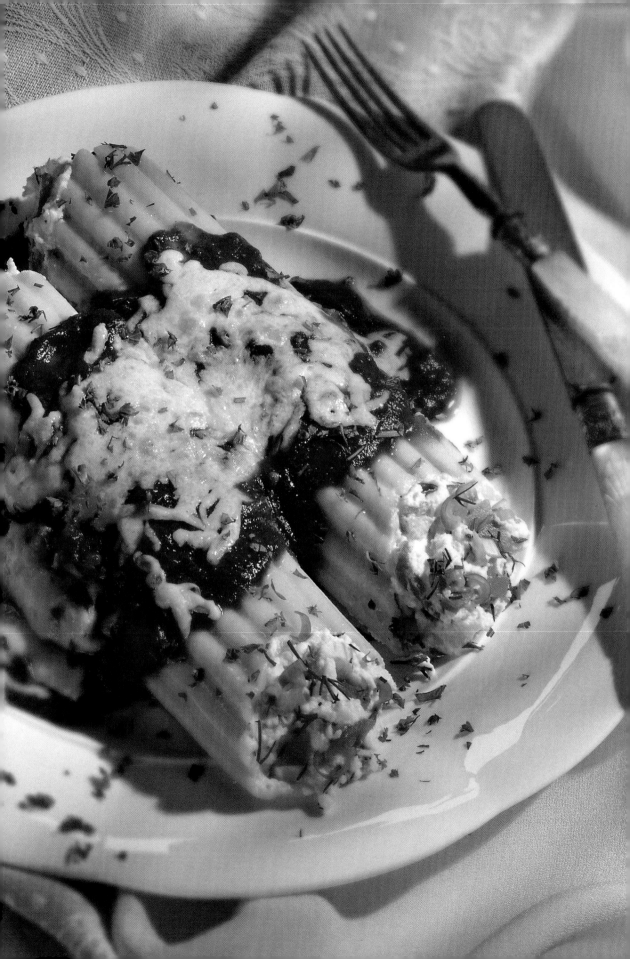

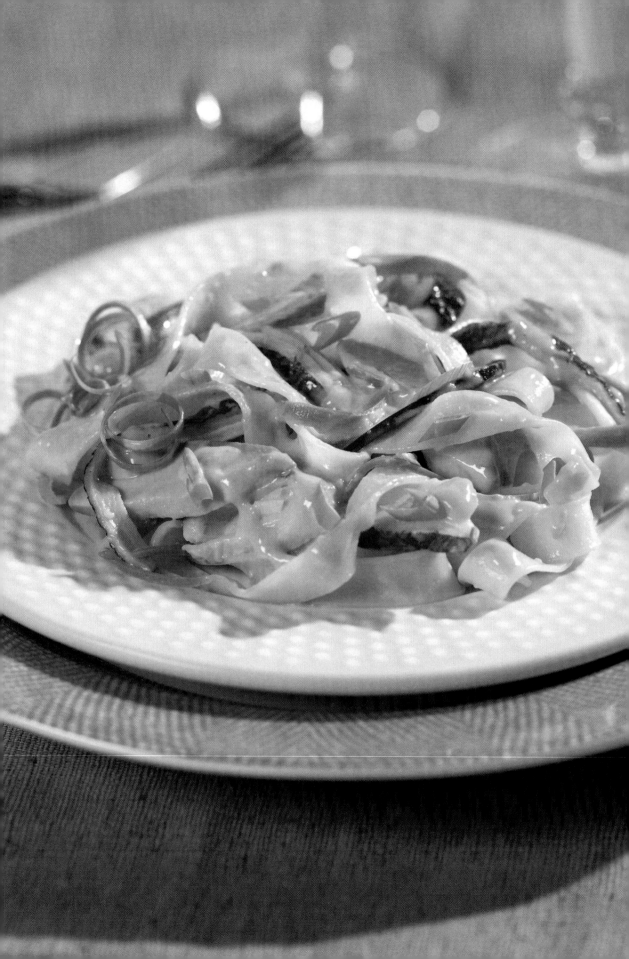

Serves 6

TIPS

Parmesan cheese can replace Asiago or Romano.

◆

Although this recipe contains 12 g of fat, the olive oil adds flavor, as well as a being a source of monounsaturated fat in the diet.

◆

Toast pine nuts in a skillet until golden brown, approximately 3 minutes.

PER SERVING		
3	■	Starch Choices
1½	◕	Fruit & Vegetable Choices
2½	◑	Protein Choices
1	▲	Fat & Oil Choice

Calories	452
Carbohydrates	62 g
Fiber	3 g
Protein	25 g
Fat, total	12 g
Fat, saturated	3 g
Sodium	768 mg
Cholesterol	35 mg

Rotini with Chicken, Sweet Peppers and Sun-Dried Tomato Sauce

12 oz	rotini	375 g
12 oz	skinless, boneless chicken breasts cut into 1-inch (2.5-cm) strips	375 g
1½ cups	thinly sliced yellow or green sweet peppers	375 mL
¼ cup	grated Asiago or Romano cheese	50 mL
SAUCE		
4 oz	sun-dried tomatoes	100 g
2 tsp	crushed garlic	10 mL
1 cup	chicken stock or water	250 mL
½ cup	chopped parsley	125 mL
2 tbsp	toasted pine nuts	25 mL
3 tbsp	olive oil	45 mL
3 tbsp	grated Parmesan cheese	45 mL

1. Cover sun-dried tomatoes with boiling water; let soak for 15 minutes. Drain and chop. Set aside.

2. Cook pasta in boiling water according to package instructions or until firm to the bite. Drain and place in serving bowl.

3. In large nonstick skillet sprayed with nonstick vegetable spray, sauté chicken until no longer pink, approximately 5 minutes. Add to pasta.

4. Respray skillet and sauté sweet peppers just until tender, approximately 4 minutes. Add to pasta with Asiago cheese.

5. Make the sauce: In food processor, combine sun-dried tomatoes, garlic, stock, parsley, nuts, oil and cheese. Purée until smooth. Pour over pasta, and toss.

MAKE AHEAD ◆ Prepare sauce up to 4 days ahead or freeze up to 4 weeks. If sauce thickens, thin with stock or water.

≺ Avocado Crab Meat over Rice Noodles (page 128)
Overleaf: Manicotti Shells Filled with Cheese and Smoked Salmon Bits (page 123)

TIP

Adjust spices according to taste. For a spicier flavor, increase cayenne.

Cajun Chicken over Fettuccine

12 oz	fettuccine	375 g
12 oz	skinless, boneless chicken breast cut into 2-inch (5-cm) strips	375 g

SPICE MIXTURE

1 tsp	cayenne	5 mL
1¾ tsp	onion powder	8 mL
1¼ tsp	garlic powder	6 mL
1 tsp	paprika	5 mL
1 tsp	dried basil	5 mL
¾ tsp	dried oregano	4 mL
2½ tbsp	unseasoned bread crumbs	35 mL

SAUCE

2 tsp	vegetable oil	10 mL
1 tsp	crushed garlic	5 mL
¾ cup	chopped onions	175 mL
¾ cup	chopped sweet green peppers	175 mL
4 cups	canned or fresh tomatoes, crushed	1 L
1½ tsp	dried basil	7 mL
1 tsp	dried oregano	5 mL
¼ tsp	cayenne	1 mL

1. Cook pasta in boiling water according to package instructions or until firm to the bite. Drain and place in serving bowl.

2. Prepare the spices: In small bowl combine cayenne, onion and garlic powders, paprika, basil, oregano and bread crumbs. Coat chicken in mixture.

3. In medium nonstick skillet sprayed with vegetable spray, sauté chicken on medium heat until no longer pink, approximately 4 minutes. Add to pasta.

continued on page 99

PER SERVING

3 ■ Starch Choices

1½ ◪ Fruit & Vegetable Choices

2 ◪ Protein Choices

Calories 379
Carbohydrates . . . . 66 g
Fiber . . . . 5 g
Protein . . . . 21 g
Fat, total . . . . 4 g
Fat, saturated . . . . . . 1 g
Sodium . . . . 462 mg
Cholesterol . . . . . 26 mg

4. Make the sauce: In same skillet, heat oil; sauté garlic, onions and green peppers for 5 minutes, until tender. Add tomatoes, basil, oregano and cayenne. Simmer for 20 to 25 minutes. Pour over pasta, and toss.

MAKE AHEAD ◆ Prepare spice mixture at any time and keep in a closed container. Coat the chicken up to a day before and refrigerate. Prepare sauce early in day. Reheat gently.

Rigatoni with Sautéed Chicken Livers in Basil Tomato Sauce

12 oz	rigatoni	375 g
1 tbsp	margarine or butter	15 mL
1½ tsp	crushed garlic	7 mL
¾ cup	diced onions	175 mL
8	medium chicken livers, cubed	8
2½ cups	canned or fresh tomatoes, crushed	625 mL
½ cup	chopped fresh basil (or 2 tsp [10 mL] dried)	125 mL
¼ cup	grated Parmesan cheese	50 mL

1. Cook pasta in boiling water according to package instructions or until firm to the bite. Drain and place in serving bowl.

2. In large nonstick skillet, melt half the margarine; sauté garlic and onions until soft, approximately 5 minutes. Sauté livers in remaining margarine just until no longer pink, approximately 5 minutes. Add tomatoes and basil; simmer on low heat for 10 minutes, stirring occasionally. Pour over pasta. Sprinkle with cheese, and toss.

MAKE AHEAD ◆ Prepare entire sauce early in day. Reheat gently, adding a little water or chicken stock if sauce thickens.

Serves 6

PER SERVING

3	■	Starch Choices
1	🥕	Fruit & Vegetable Choice
1½	◎	Protein Choices
½	▲	Fat & Oil Choice

Calories 361
Carbohydrates . . . . 58 g
Fiber . . . . 3 g
Protein . . . . 19 g
Fat, total . . . . 6 g
Fat, saturated . . . . 2 g
Sodium . . . . 391 mg
Cholesterol . . . . 191 mg

Chicken Tetrazzini

TIPS

Try this dish with macaroni or penne instead of spaghetti.

◆

Substitute fresh tuna or swordfish for the chicken.

◆

Substituting low-fat cheddar cheese (20% m.f.) for regular cheddar will reduce the fat content of this recipe by 3 g and saturated fat by 2 g/serving.

◆

Substitute the chicken with 4 oz (125 g) of cooked seafood for a change.

8 oz	spaghetti	250 g
4 tsp	margarine	20 mL
1½ tsp	crushed garlic	7 mL
1 cup	chopped onion	250 mL
1 cup	chopped sweet red pepper	250 mL
1 cup	sliced mushrooms	250 mL
3 tbsp	all-purpose flour	45 mL
1½ cups	chicken stock	375 mL
1 cup	2% milk	250 mL
3 tbsp	white wine	45 mL
1½ tsp	Dijon mustard	7 mL
4 oz	cooked boneless skinless chicken pieces	125 g
½ cup	shredded Cheddar cheese	125 mL
1 tbsp	grated Parmesan cheese Chopped fresh parsley	15 mL

1. In saucepan of boiling water, cook spaghetti according to package directions or until firm to the bite; drain.

2. Meanwhile, in nonstick saucepan, melt margarine; sauté garlic, onion, red pepper and mushrooms until softened, approximately 5 minutes. Add flour and cook, stirring, for 1 minute.

3. Add stock, milk, wine and mustard; cook, stirring, for 3 minutes or until thickened. Add chicken.

4. Add sauce to spaghetti and toss to mix well; place in baking dish. Sprinkle Cheddar and Parmesan cheeses over top; bake until top is golden, approximately 5 minutes. Garnish with parsley.

PER SERVING

2 ■ Starch Choices

1 ◆ Fruit & Vegetable Choice

2 ◉ Protein Choices

1½ ▲ Fat & Oil Choices

Calories 355

Carbohydrates . . . . 40 g

Fiber . . . . 2 g

Protein . . . . 18 g

Fat, total . . . . 12 g

Fat, saturated . . . . 6 g

Sodium . . . . 603 mg

Cholesterol . . . . . 34 mg

Serve this salad with whole grain bread and complete the meal with a ½ cup (125 mL) of no sugar added fruit yogurt served over sliced pears or orange sections.

◆

Substitute broccoli or fresh green beans for the asparagus.

Chicken and Asparagus Salad
with Lemon Dill Vinaigrette

12	baby red potatoes (or 4 small white)	12
8 oz	boneless skinless chicken breasts, cubed	250 g
¼ cup	water	50 mL
¼ cup	white wine	50 mL
8 oz	asparagus, trimmed and cut into small pieces	250 g
2	small heads Boston lettuce, torn into pieces	2

LEMON DILL VINAIGRETTE

3 tbsp	balsamic vinegar	45 mL
2 tbsp	lemon juice	25 mL
I tbsp	water	15 mL
I large	green onion, minced	I
¾ tsp	garlic	4 mL
2 tbsp	chopped fresh dill (or I tsp [5 mL] dried dillweed)	25 mL
3 tbsp	olive oil	45 mL

I. In saucepan of boiling water, cook potatoes until just tender. Peel and cut into cubes. Place in salad bowl and set aside.

2. In saucepan, bring chicken, water and wine to boil; reduce heat, cover and simmer for approximately 2 minutes or until chicken is no longer pink. Drain and add to potatoes in bowl.

3. Steam or microwave asparagus until just tender-crisp; drain and add to bowl. Add lettuce.

4. Lemon Dill Vinaigrette: In bowl, whisk together vinegar, lemon juice, water, onion, garlic and dill; whisk in oil until combined. Pour over chicken mixture; toss to coat well.

PER SERVING

I	■ Starch Choice
I	◉ Protein Choice
I	▲ Fat & Oil Choice
I	✣ Extra Choice

Calories 186
Carbohydrates . . . . 19 g
Fiber . . . . 2 g
Protein . . . . 10 g
Fat, total . . . . 8 g
Fat, saturated . . . . I g
Sodium . . . . 24 mg
Cholesterol . . . . . 18 mg

Great combination of
ratatouille and chili in
one dish.

◆

Great as a family meal.
Serve with French bread.

◆

Ground pork, veal
or chicken can
replace turkey.

Turkey Ratatouille Chili

2 tsp	vegetable oil	10 mL
2 tsp	minced garlic	10 mL
1 cup	chopped onions	250 mL
1⅔ cups	chopped zucchini	400 mL
1⅔ cups	chopped peeled eggplant	400 mL
1½ cups	chopped mushrooms	375 mL
12 oz	ground turkey	375 g
2 tbsp	tomato paste	25 mL
1	can (19 oz [540 mL]) tomatoes, puréed	1
2 cups	chicken stock	500 mL
1⅓ cups	peeled chopped potatoes	325 mL
1 cup	canned red kidney beans, drained	250 mL
1 tbsp	chili powder	15 mL
1½ tsp	dried basil	7 mL
1	bay leaf	1

1. In large nonstick saucepan sprayed with vegetable spray, heat oil over medium heat. Add garlic, onions, zucchini and eggplant; cook for 5 minutes or until softened. Add mushrooms and cook 2 minutes longer. Remove vegetables from skillet and set aside. Add turkey to skillet and cook for 3 minutes, stirring to break it up, or until no longer pink. Drain fat and add cooked vegetables to skillet.

2. Add tomato paste, tomatoes, stock, potatoes, beans, chili powder, basil and bay leaf; bring to a boil. Cover, reduce heat to low and simmer for 40 minutes, stirring occasionally.

MAKE AHEAD ◆ Prepare up to a day ahead and reheat gently, adding extra chicken stock if too thick.

PER SERVING

1	■	Starch Choice
1½	◢	Fruit & Vegetable Choices
2½	◢	Protein Choices

Calories 250
Carbohydrates . . . . 36 g
Fiber . . . . 7 g
Protein . . . . 20 g
Fat, total . . . . 4 g
Fat, saturated . . . . 1 g
Sodium . . . . 615 mg
Cholesterol . . . . . 37 mg

Meat

There are many ◉ Protein choices which can balance a meal. Meat is one tasty choice that forms the staple of many main entrées. Today's meat is much leaner than before. Meat is also great source of iron and nutrients. In fact, the iron in meat called "heme" iron is absorbed more readily by the body than iron found in other sources. Always choose lean cuts of meat, trimmed of fat, as they will contain less total fat and saturated fat.

❖

Steak Kabobs
with Honey Garlic Marinade

2 tbsp	soya sauce	25 mL
2 tbsp	sherry or rice vinegar	25 mL
4 tsp	honey	20 mL
2 tsp	crushed garlic	10 mL
1½ tsp	sesame oil	7 mL
4 tsp	vegetable oil	20 mL
1 tbsp	water	15 mL
¾ lb	lean steak, cut into cubes	375 g
16	pieces (1-inch [2.5cm]) sweet green pepper	16
16	pieces (1-inch [2.5cm]) onion	16
16	small mushrooms	16
16	snow peas	16

1. In bowl, combine soya sauce, sherry, honey, garlic, sesame and vegetable oils and water. Add steak and marinate for 30 minutes, or longer in refrigerator.

2. Remove beef from marinade. Place marinade in small saucepan and cook for 3 to 5 minutes or until thick and syrupy.

3. Thread beef, green pepper, onion, mushrooms and snow peas alternately onto 8 metal skewers. Place on greased grill and barbecue for 10 to 15 minutes, turning often and brushing with marinade, or until cooked as desired. Serve with any remaining marinade.

MAKE AHEAD ◆ If possible, marinate overnight to enhance the flavor of the steak. Turn occasionally. Leftover marinade can be used as part of the liquid to cook plain rice, which is then served with the Kabobs.

PER SERVING

1½ ◑ Fruit & Vegetable Choices

½ ✳ Sugar Choice

3 ◑ Protein Choices

Calories	252
Carbohydrates	22 g
Fiber	3 g
Protein	24 g
Fat, total	9 g
Fat, saturated	1 g
Sodium	541 mg
Cholesterol	37 mg

Serve with rice noodles, instead of traditional pasta. Complete meal with a no sugar added fruit flavored yogurt.

◆

Look for a large iceberg lettuce to get the best quality leaves.

◆

Use other vegetables such as celery and oyster mushrooms as substitutes.

Oriental Beef Bundles in Lettuce

12 oz	lean ground beef	375 g
SAUCE		
2 tbsp	hoisin sauce	25 mL
1 tbsp	rice wine vinegar	15 mL
2 tsp	minced garlic	10 mL
1½ tsp	minced gingerroot	7 mL
1 tsp	sesame oil	5 mL
1 tsp	vegetable oil	5 mL
⅓ cup	finely chopped carrots	75 mL
¾ cup	finely chopped red or green peppers	175 mL
¾ cup	finely chopped mushrooms	175 mL
½ cup	chopped water chestnuts	125 mL
2	green onions, chopped	2
2 tbsp	hoisin sauce	25 mL
1 tbsp	water	15 mL
8	large iceberg lettuce leaves	8

1. Sauce: In small bowl, whisk together hoisin, vinegar, garlic, gingerroot and sesame oil; set aside.

2. In nonstick skillet sprayed with vegetable spray, cook beef over medium heat for 5 minutes, or until browned; remove from skillet. Drain any excess liquid.

3. In same nonstick skillet, heat oil over medium heat. Add carrots and cook for 3 minutes. Add red peppers and mushrooms and cook for 3 minutes or until softened. Return beef to pan along with water chestnuts and green onions. Add sauce and cook for 2 minutes.

4. Combine hoisin sauce and water in small bowl. Place a little over leaves. Divide beef mixture among lettuce leaves. Serve open or rolled up.

MAKE AHEAD ◆ Prepare entire beef mixture earlier in the day. Reheat gently before placing in lettuce leaves.

PER SERVING

1	◧	Fruit & Vegetable Choice
½	✳	Sugar Choices
2½	◕	Protein Choices
2	▲	Fat & Oil Choices

Calories 301
Carbohydrates . . . . 16 g
Fiber . . . . 2 g
Protein . . . . 20 g
Fat, total . . . . 17 g
Fat, saturated . . . . 6 g
Sodium . . . . 302 mg
Cholesterol . . . . . 53 mg

Hoisin sauce can be found in Chinese food section of the grocery store.

◆

Use any lean steak such as rib eye, porterhouse or filet tenderloin.

◆

Hoisin sauce is a sweet sauce made from flour, soybeans, chili, red beans and vegetables. Although it adds ½ ✳ Sugar choice to each portion, the recipe, the wonderful flavor it lends is well worth it.

PER SERVING

3	▣	Starch Choices
½	◪	Fruit & Vegetable Choice
½	✳	Sugar Choice
2	◪	Protein Choices
1	✦✦	Extra Choice

Calories	382
Carbohydrates	61 g
Fiber	3 g
Protein	20 g
Fat, total	6 g
Fat, saturated	1 g
Sodium	657 mg
Cholesterol	21 mg

Hoisin Beef, Red Peppers and Snow Peas over Fettuccine

12 oz	fettuccine	375 g
2 tsp	crushed garlic	10 mL
12 oz	sirloin steak cut into ½-inch (1-cm) strips	375 g
2 tsp	vegetable oil	10 mL
1 cup	thinly sliced sweet red peppers	250 mL
1 cup	snow peas, cut in half	250 mL
6 oz	sliced mushrooms	150 g
⅓ cup	chopped green onions	75 mL
¼ cup	sliced water chestnuts	50 mL

SAUCE

¾ cup	cold beef stock	175 mL
¼ cup	hoisin sauce	50 mL
2 tbsp	soya sauce	25 mL
1 tbsp	rice wine vinegar	15 mL
1 tbsp	cornstarch	15 mL
2 tsp	sesame oil	10 mL
2 tsp	minced gingerroot	10 mL

1. Cook pasta in boiling water according to package instructions or until firm to the bite. Drain and place in serving bowl.

2. Make the sauce: In small bowl, combine stock, hoisin sauce, soya sauce, rice wine vinegar, cornstarch, oil and gingerroot. Stir until smooth. Set aside.

3. In large nonstick skillet sprayed with vegetable spray, sauté garlic and steak just until beef is barely cooked, approximately 3 minutes. Drain and set beef aside.

continued on page 107

4. In same skillet, heat oil; add red peppers and snow peas; sauté for 2 minutes. Add mushrooms, green onions and water chestnuts; sauté for 3 minutes. Add sauce and beef and simmer on medium heat until sauce thickens slightly, for 3 or 4 minutes, stirring constantly. Pour over pasta, and toss.

MAKE AHEAD ◆ Prepare sauce up to a day ahead, stirring before use.

Serves 4 or 5

Start barbecue or preheat oven to 450°F (230°C)

TIPS

Ground chicken or veal can replace beef.

◆

Serve these burgers on a kaiser roll or pita bun.

Hoisin Garlic Burgers

I lb	lean ground beef	500 g
¼ cup	bread crumbs	50 mL
¼ cup	chopped green onions (about 2 medium)	50 mL
3 tbsp	chopped coriander or parsley	45 mL
2 tbsp	hoisin sauce	25 mL
2 tsp	minced garlic	10 mL
I tsp	minced gingerroot	5 mL
I	egg	I
2 tbsp	water	25 mL
2 tbsp	hoisin sauce	25 mL
I tsp	sesame oil	5 mL

I. In bowl combine beef, bread crumbs, green onions, coriander, hoisin sauce, garlic, gingerroot and egg; mix well. Make 4 to 5 burgers.

2. In small bowl whisk together water, hoisin sauce and sesame oil. Brush half of the sauce over top of burgers.

3. Place on greased grill and barbecue, or place on rack on baking sheet and bake for 10 to 15 minutes (or until no longer pink inside). Turn patties once and brush with remaining sauce.

MAKE AHEAD ◆ Prepare beef mixture up to a day ahead and form into burgers. Freeze up to 6 weeks.

PER SERVING

I	✳ Sugar Choice
3	◑ Protein Choices
I½	▲ Fat & Oil Choices

Calories 292
Carbohydrates . . . . 10 g
Fiber . . . . I g
Protein . . . . 21 g
Fat, total . . . . 18 g
Fat, saturated . . . . 7 g
Sodium . . . . 305 mg
Cholesterol . . . . 100 mg

Children love this version of packaged Beefaroni. It is not only more delicious, it is healthier for them.

◆

Double this recipe and serve it to a group.

◆

Substitute ground chicken or veal for the beef.

Beef, Macaroni and Cheese Casserole

1 ½ tsp	vegetable oil	7 mL
2 tsp	crushed garlic	10 mL
½ cup	chopped onion	125 mL
12 oz	lean ground beef	375 g
1	can (19 oz [540 mL]) tomatoes, crushed	1
1 tsp	dried basil	5 mL
1 tsp	dried oregano	5 mL
1 cup	macaroni	250 mL
2 tbsp	grated Parmesan cheese	25 mL

1. In large nonstick skillet, heat oil; sauté garlic and onion for 3 minutes. Add beef and sauté until no longer pink, stirring constantly to break up beef.

2. Add tomatoes, basil and oregano; cover and cook for 15 minutes, stirring occasionally.

3. Meanwhile, cook macaroni according to package directions or until firm to the bite. Drain and place in serving bowl. Toss with sauce and sprinkle with cheese.

MAKE AHEAD ◆ Cook and refrigerate up to a day before, then reheat to serve.

PER SERVING

1 ½ ■ Starch Choices

½ ◨ Fruit & Vegetable Choice

3 ◉ Protein Choices

1 ½ ▲ Fat & Oil Choices

1 ◆◆ Extra Choice

Calories 383
Carbohydrates . . . . 33 g
Fiber . . . . 3 g
Protein . . . . 24 g
Fat, total . . . . 18 g
Fat, saturated . . . . 7 g
Sodium . . . . 485 mg
Cholesterol . . . . . 55 mg

Pizza Pasta with Beef-Tomato Sauce and Cheese

6 oz	macaroni	150 g
1	egg	1
⅓ cup	2% milk	75 mL
3 tbsp	grated Parmesan cheese	45 mL
1 tsp	vegetable oil	5 mL
2 tsp	crushed garlic	10 mL
¾ cup	finely chopped onions	175 mL
½ cup	finely chopped sweet green peppers	125 mL
⅓ cup	finely chopped carrots	75 mL
8 oz	ground beef or chicken	250 g
1	can (19 oz [540 mL]) tomatoes, crushed	1
2 tbsp	tomato paste	25 mL
1½ tsp	dried basil	7 mL
1 tsp	dried oregano	5 mL
1 cup	low-fat mozzarella cheese, shredded	250 mL

1. Cook pasta in boiling water according to package instructions or until firm to the bite. Drain and place in serving bowl. Add egg, milk and cheese. Mix well. Place in baking pan as a crust and bake for 20 minutes.

2. Meanwhile, in medium nonstick saucepan sprayed with vegetable spray, heat oil; sauté garlic, onions, green peppers and carrots until tender, approximately 5 minutes. Add beef and sauté until no longer pink, approximately 4 minutes. Add tomatoes, tomato paste, basil and oregano. Cover and simmer on low heat for 15 minutes, stirring occasionally.

3. Pour sauce into pasta crust. Sprinkle with cheese; bake for 10 minutes or until cheese melts.

MAKE AHEAD ◆ Prepare pasta crust and sauce early in day. Store separately.

Serves 4

Preheat oven to 400°F
(200°C)

PER SERVING

½ ◢ Fruit & Vegetable
    Choice

4½ ◢ Protein Choices

Calories	266
Carbohydrates	7 g
Fiber	1 g
Protein	33 g
Fat, total	11 g
Fat, saturated	4 g
Sodium	559 mg
Cholesterol	111 mg

Veal Stuffed with Cheese in Mushroom Sauce

1 lb	veal cutlets	500 g
1 tsp	vegetable oil	5 mL
½ cup	finely diced mushrooms	125 mL
¼ cup	finely diced onions	50 mL
1 tsp	crushed garlic	5 mL
⅓ cup	shredded mozzarella cheese	75 mL
¼ cup	beef stock	50 mL
	Chopped fresh parsley	

SAUCE

1 tbsp	margarine	15 mL
1½ cups	sliced mushrooms	375 mL
2 tbsp	all-purpose flour	25 mL
1 cup	beef stock	250 mL
1 tbsp	sherry (optional)	15 mL
2 tbsp	light sour cream	25 mL

1. Pound veal until flat and divide into 4 serving pieces.

2. In small nonstick skillet, heat oil; sauté mushrooms, onions and garlic until softened, approximately 3 minutes. Remove from heat.

3. Divide vegetable mixture among cutlets. Sprinkle cheese over top. Roll up and secure with toothpick. Place in baking dish and add stock. Cover and bake for 8 to 10 minutes or just until veal is tender. Remove rolls to serving platter. Keep warm.

4. Sauce: In small nonstick skillet, melt margarine; sauté mushrooms until softened and liquid is released. Add flour and cook, stirring, for 1 minute. Add stock, and sherry (if using); cook until thickened, approximately 2 minutes, stirring constantly. If too thick, add more stock. Remove from heat and stir in sour cream; pour over veal. Garnish with parsley.

MAKE AHEAD ◆ Assemble and refrigerate veal rolls early in the day. Make sauce ahead of time but add sour cream after reheating.

TIPS

Chicken can be substituted for the veal.

◆

Adjust the chili powder to your taste.

◆

Serve on a bed of rice or pasta and steamed broccoli or green beans on the side. Complete the meal with Frozen Vanilla Yogurt (page 181).

Spicy Veal Meatballs
with Tomato Sauce

12 oz	ground veal	375 g
¼ cup	finely chopped onion	50 mL
2 tsp	crushed garlic	10 mL
¼ cup	finely chopped sweet red pepper	50 mL
1	egg	1
1½ tsp	grated Parmesan cheese	7 mL
⅓ cup	dry bread crumbs	75 mL
2 tbsp	chili sauce or ketchup	25 mL
2 tbsp	chopped fresh basil (or 1 tsp [5 mL] dried)	25 mL
1 tsp	chili powder	5 mL
1¾ cups	tomato sauce, heated	425 mL

1. In large bowl, mix together veal, onion, garlic, red pepper, egg, cheese, bread crumbs, chili sauce, basil and chili powder until well combined. Roll into 1-inch (2.5 cm) balls and place on baking sheet.

2. Bake for approximately 10 minutes or until no longer pink inside. Place in serving dish and pour tomato sauce over top.

MAKE AHEAD ◆ Prepare and refrigerate meatballs up to a day before serving, then reheat on low temperature.

PER SERVING		
1	■ Starch Choice	
2	◐ Protein Choices	
1	✚✚ Extra Choice	

Calories	172
Carbohydrates	14 g
Fiber	2 g
Protein	16 g
Fat, total	6 g
Fat, saturated	2 g
Sodium	589 mg
Cholesterol	88 mg

Use chicken, pork or turkey scallopini to replace veal.

◆

Use frozen pineapple juice concentrate and replace remainder in freezer. Orange juice can also be used.

◆

If limes are unavailable, use lemons.

Veal with Pineapple Lime Sauce and Pecans

I lb	veal scallopini	500 g
2 tsp	oil	10 mL
3 tbsp	flour	45 mL
SAUCE		
¼ cup	chopped green onions (about 2 medium)	50 mL
2 tbsp	chopped pecans	25 mL
¼ cup	pineapple juice concentrate	50 mL
¼ cup	water	50 mL
I tbsp	honey	15 mL
I tbsp	fresh lime juice	15 mL
I tsp	grated lime zest	5 mL

I. Between sheets of waxed paper pound veal to ¼-inch (5-mm) thickness. In large nonstick skillet sprayed with vegetable spray, heat oil over medium-high heat. Dredge veal in flour and cook for 2½ minutes per side or until just done at center. Place on a serving dish and cover.

2. Add green onions and pecans to skillet. Cook for 2 minutes. Add pineapple juice concentrate, water, honey, lime juice and lime zest. Bring to a boil for 1 minute, or until slightly syrupy and thickened. Serve sauce over veal.

MAKE AHEAD ◆ Prepare sauce earlier in the day and reheat gently before serving. Add more water if too thick.

PER SERVING

1½ ◨ Fruit & Vegetable Choices

½ ✳ Sugar Choice

2 ◨ Protein Choices

Calories	210
Carbohydrates	19 g
Fiber	1 g
Protein	18 g
Fat, total	7 g
Fat, saturated	1 g
Sodium	68 mg
Cholesterol	67 mg

Use beef steak or boneless chicken breast instead of pork.

◆

Serve over pasta or rice. This recipe is high in carbohydrate when compared to most other meat entrées. Using a granulated sugar substitute in the place of the brown sugar may alter the taste slightly, but will reduce the total carbohydrate content to 20 g/serving and the ✳ Sugars choice to ½.

PER SERVING

1½ 🍎 Fruit & Vegetable Choices

2 ✳ Sugar Choices

3 🔶 Protein Choices

Calories 291
Carbohydrates . . . . 37 g
Fiber . . . . 3 g
Protein . . . . 22 g
Fat, total . . . . 7 g
Fat, saturated . . . . 2 g
Sodium . . . . 862 mg
Cholesterol . . . . . 55 mg

Pork Stir-Fry
with Sweet and Sour Sauce, Snow Peas and Red Peppers

SAUCE

1 cup	chicken stock	250 mL
⅓ cup	brown sugar	75 mL
⅓ cup	ketchup	75 mL
2 tbsp	rice wine vinegar	25 mL
1 tbsp	soya sauce	15 mL
2 tsp	sesame oil	10 mL
4 tsp	cornstarch	20 mL
2 tsp	minced garlic	10 mL
1½ tsp	minced gingerroot	7 mL
12 oz	pork loin, cut into thin strips	375 g
1 tsp	vegetable oil	5 mL
1½ cups	snow peas or sugar snap peas	375 mL
1¼ cups	red pepper strips	300 mL
¾ cup	green pepper strips	175 mL
½ cup	chopped green onions (about 4 medium)	125 mL

1. In small bowl combine stock, brown sugar, ketchup, vinegar, soya sauce, sesame oil, cornstarch, garlic and ginger; set aside.

2. In nonstick wok or skillet sprayed with vegetable spray, cook the pork strips over high heat for 2 minutes, stirring constantly, or until just done at center; remove from wok.

3. Add oil to wok. Cook snow peas, red and green peppers for 3 minutes, stirring constantly, or until tender-crisp. Stir sauce again and add to wok along with pork. Cook for 45 seconds or until thickened. Garnish with green onions.

MAKE AHEAD ◆ Prepare sauce up to a day before.

Preheat oven to 425°F (220°C)

Baking sheet sprayed with vegetable spray

TIPS

Use pork chops or pork cutlets or substitute boneless chicken or beef steak. Mozzarella cheese can replace Cheddar.

◆

If you use low-fat cheese the total fat will be 14 g with only 6 g of saturated fat and the ▲ Fat & Oil Choices will be reduced to ½.

PER SERVING

1	■	Starch Choice
1½	◢	Fruit & Vegetable Choices
3½	◉	Protein Choices
1½	▲	Fat & Oil Choices

Calories 405
Carbohydrates . . . . 33 g
Fiber . . . . 4 g
Protein . . . . 27 g
Fat, total . . . . 19 g
Fat, saturated . . . . . . 9 g
Sodium . . . . 434 mg
Cholesterol . . . . . 72 mg

Pork Fajitas
with Sweet Peppers, Coriander and Cheese

8 oz	pork tenderloin, cut into thin strips	250 g
2 tsp	vegetable oil	10 mL
1½ tsp	minced garlic	7 mL
1½ cups	thinly sliced onions	375 mL
1½ cups	red pepper strips	375 mL
¼ cup	fresh chopped coriander or parsley	50 mL
3 tbsp	chopped green onions (about 2 medium)	45 mL
4	large flour tortillas	4
½ cup	grated Cheddar cheese	125 mL
⅓ cup	bottled salsa	75 mL
¼ cup	light sour cream	50 mL

1. In nonstick skillet sprayed with vegetable spray, cook the pork strips over high heat for 2 minutes, or until just done at center. Remove from skillet. Add oil. Cook garlic and onions for 4 minutes until browned. Add red pepper strips and cook over medium heat for 5 minutes, or until softened.

2. Remove from heat and stir in coriander, green onions and pork. Divide among tortillas. Top with Cheddar, salsa and sour cream. Roll up, place on baking sheet and bake for 5 minutes or until heated through.

MAKE AHEAD ◆ Prepare pork mixture earlier in the day. Reheat gently and fill tortillas.

Preheat oven to 375°F
(190°C)

TIPS

Lamb can be butterflied
and filled, then gently
folded over and tied
with a string.

◆

Complete this meal with
a simple dessert of fresh
fruit topped with ½ cup
(125 mL) of fat-free no
sugar added vanilla
pudding. If your meal
plan allows additional
■ Starch choices add a
couple of plain cookies.

PER SERVING

1½ ■ Starch Choices
½ ◢ Fruit & Vegetable
    Choice
3½ ◢ Protein Choices

Calories 335
Carbohydrates . . . . 30 g
Fiber . . . . 2 g
Protein . . . . 28 g
Fat, total . . . . 10 g
Fat, saturated . . . . 3 g
Sodium . . . . 704 mg
Cholesterol . . . . . 72 mg

Leg of Lamb
with Pesto and Wild Rice

STUFFING

1 tsp	vegetable oil	5 mL
2 tsp	minced garlic	10 mL
1 cup	chopped onions	250 mL
1 cup	chopped red or green peppers	250 mL
¾ cup	wild rice	175 mL
¾ cup	white rice	175 mL
3 cups	beef or chicken stock	750 mL
⅓ cup	pesto (see recipe, page 163)	75 mL
3 lb	boneless leg of lamb with a pocket	1.5 kg
1 tsp	vegetable oil	5 mL
1 tsp	minced garlic	5 mL
⅔ cup	beef stock	150 mL
½ cup	red or white wine	125 mL

1. In saucepan, heat oil over medium heat. Add garlic and onions and cook for 3 minutes or until softened. Add red peppers and cook for 2 minutes longer. Add rices and cook, stirring, for 3 minutes. Add stock; bring to a boil, cover, reduce heat to medium-low and simmer covered for 20 to 25 minutes or until rice is tender and liquid absorbed. Stir in pesto. Set aside to cool.

2. Stuff leg of lamb with some of the cooled rice mixture; put leftover stuffing in a casserole dish and cover. Rub lamb with oil and garlic and place on rack in roasting pan. Truss lamb with string. Pour stock and wine under lamb. Bake covered for 20 minutes, basting with pan juices every 10 minutes. Uncover lamb and bake another 20 to 25 minutes, basting every 10 minutes. Add extra stock if liquids evaporate. Put casserole dish with leftover stuffing in the oven for the last 20 minutes. Serve meat with juices.

MAKE AHEAD ◆ Prepare pesto up to 2 days before and keep refrigerated. Can also be frozen for up to 4 weeks.

Serves 4

Curried Lamb Casserole
with Sweet Potatoes

¾ lb	lamb, cut into ¾-inch (2 cm) cubes	375 g
	All-purpose flour for dusting	
1 tbsp	vegetable oil	15 mL
2 tsp	crushed garlic	10 mL
1 cup	chopped onion	250 mL
1 cup	finely chopped carrots	250 mL
½ cup	finely chopped sweet green pepper	125 mL
1 cup	cubed peeled sweet potatoes	250 mL
1½ cups	sliced mushrooms	375 mL
2½ cups	beef stock	625 mL
⅓ cup	red wine	75 mL
3 tbsp	tomato paste	45 mL
2 tsp	curry powder	10 mL

1. Dust lamb with flour.

2. In large nonstick Dutch oven, heat oil, sauté lamb for 2 minutes or just until seared all over. Remove lamb and set aside.

3. To skillet, add garlic, onion, carrots, green pepper and sweet potatoes; cook, stirring often, for 8 to 10 minutes or until tender. Add mushrooms and cook until softened, approximately 3 minutes.

4. Add stock, wine, tomato paste and curry powder. Return lamb to pan; cover and simmer for 1½ hours, stirring occasionally.

MAKE AHEAD ◆ Make and refrigerate up to a day ahead and reheat on low heat. This dish can also be frozen.

PER SERVING

1	■	Starch Choice
1	◢	Fruit & Vegetable Choice
3	◙	Protein Choices

Calories 310
Carbohydrates . . . . 32 g
Fiber . . . . 5 g
Protein . . . . 23 g
Fat, total . . . . 9 g
Fat, saturated . . . . 2 g
Sodium . . . . 783 mg
Cholesterol . . . . . 61 mg

Pasta and Grains

All pasta sold in Canada is now fortified with folic acid so most of the recipes containing pasta will be a good source of this nutrient. You can also increase the fiber content of the pasta recipes by looking for whole grain pastas in your supermarket.

Combined with ◧ Fruit & Vegetable Choices and with small amounts of food from the ◉ Protein Choices, many of these recipes are almost complete meals in themselves. Check your meal plan to include any missing choices.

Pasta and grains provide the foundation of many diets. Using the Good Health Eating Guide system, pasta and grains are ■ Starch choices and ½ cup (125 mL) of cooked pasta or grain is usually 1 Starch.

❖

For a less distinct basil flavor, use half parsley and half basil.

♦

Toast pine nuts on top of stove in skillet until brown, for 2 to 3 minutes.

Linguine with Pesto Chicken

12 oz	linguine	375 g
12 oz	skinless, boneless chicken breasts, thinly sliced	375 g

SAUCE

2 cups	fresh basil, packed down	500 mL
⅓ cup	chicken stock	75 mL
3 tbsp	olive oil	45 mL
2 tbsp	grated Parmesan cheese	25 mL
2 tbsp	toasted pine nuts or walnuts	25 mL
1½ tsp	crushed garlic	7 mL

1. Cook pasta in boiling water according to package instructions or until firm to the bite. Drain and place in serving bowl.

2. In medium nonstick skillet sprayed with vegetable spray, sauté chicken until no longer pink, approximately 3 minutes. Add to pasta.

3. Make the sauce: In food processor, purée basil, stock, oil, cheese, nuts and garlic until smooth. Pour over pasta, and toss.

MAKE AHEAD ♦ Refrigerate sauce for up to 5 days or up to 3 weeks in freezer.

PER SERVING

3	■ Starch Choices
2	◗ Protein Choices
1	▲ Fat & Oil Choice

Calories 373
Carbohydrates . . . . 48 g
Fiber . . . . 2 g
Protein . . . . 20 g
Fat, total . . . . 11 g
Fat, saturated . . . . 2 g
Sodium . . . . 121 mg
Cholesterol . . . . . 27 mg

As a substitute for the turkey, try using ground veal, beef or chicken.

◆

This meal is an excellent source of vitamin C, B$_6$, niacin, folate, magnesium and a good source of phosphorus, iron, zinc, niacin and vitamin A.

Pasta with Spicy Turkey Tomato Sauce

12 oz	rotini	375 g
2 tsp	vegetable oil	10 mL
2 tsp	crushed garlic	10 mL
1 cup	diced red onions	250 mL
1 cup	diced red or green peppers	250 mL
12 oz	ground turkey	375 g
3 cups	crushed tomatoes (canned or fresh)	750 mL
1 ½ tsp	dried basil	7 mL
1 tsp	dried oregano	5 mL
2 tsp	chili powder	10 mL
Pinch	cayenne pepper	Pinch
½ cup	coriander leaves or parsley, chopped	125 mL

1. Cook pasta in boiling water according to package instructions or until firm to the bite. Drain and place in serving bowl.

2. In large nonstick saucepan sprayed with vegetable spray, heat oil; sauté garlic, onions and red peppers until soft, approximately 5 minutes. Add turkey and sauté on medium heat until cooked, approximately 5 minutes.

3. Add tomatoes, basil, oregano, chili powder and cayenne. Cover and simmer on low heat for 15 minutes, stirring occasionally. Add coriander. Pour over pasta, and toss.

MAKE AHEAD ◆ Sauce can be prepared up to 2 days before and gently reheated before serving. Do not add coriander or parsley until ready to serve.

PER SERVING

2½ ■ Starch Choices

1 ◗ Fruit & Vegetable Choice

2 ◉ Protein Choices

1 ✦✦ Extra Choice

Calories 342
Carbohydrates . . . . 54 g
Fiber . . . . 4 g
Protein . . . . 22 g
Fat, total . . . . 5 g
Fat, saturated . . . . 1 g
Sodium . . . . 63 mg
Cholesterol . . . . . 37 mg

A granulated sugar substitute can replace the brown sugar in this recipe and eliminate the ½ ✱ Sugars choice or save about 5 g of carbohydrate/serving.

◆

Sodium or salt content of this recipe can be reduced by using a low-sodium soy sauce.

Rotini with Stir-Fried Steak and Crisp Vegetables

½ lb	rotini	250 g
1 ½ tsp	vegetable oil	7 mL
1 cup	diced onions	250 mL
1 cup	chopped broccoli	250 mL
1 cup	snow peas	250 mL
½ cup	diced carrots	125 mL
8 oz	steak, sliced thinly	250 g
½ cup	sliced water chestnuts	125 mL

SAUCE

½ cup	hot water	125 mL
¼ cup	soya sauce	50 mL
2 tbsp	brown sugar	25 mL
2 ½ tsp	cornstarch	12 mL
1 ½ tsp	grated gingerroot (or ½ tsp [2 mL] ground ginger)	7 mL
1 tsp	crushed garlic	5 mL

1. Sauce: In small bowl, combine water, soya sauce, sugar, cornstarch, ginger and garlic; set aside.

2. Cook rotini according to package directions or until firm to the bite. Drain and place in serving bowl.

3. Meanwhile, in nonstick skillet, heat oil; sauté onions, broccoli, snow peas and carrots almost until tendercrisp, approximately 5 minutes.

4. Add steak and water chestnuts; sauté for 1 minute. Add sauce; cook, stirring, just until beef is cooked, approximately 2 minutes. Pour over pasta and mix well.

MAKE AHEAD ◆ Make sauce early in day and add steak to marinate in refrigerator until cooking time.

PER SERVING

2½ ▣ Starch Choices

1 ◢ Fruit & Vegetable Choice

½ ✱ Sugar Choice

2 ◭ Protein Choices

Calories 343
Carbohydrates . . . . 57 g
Fiber . . . . 4 g
Protein . . . . 20 g
Fat, total . . . . 3 g
Fat, saturated . . . . 1 g
Sodium . . . . 828 mg
Cholesterol . . . . . 20 mg

This is delicious served
warm or cold.

◆

The goat cheese can
be substituted with
feta cheese.

Rotini with Tomatoes, Black Olives and Goat Cheese

I tbsp	vegetable oil	15 mL
I ½ tsp	crushed garlic	7 mL
I cup	chopped onions	250 mL
I	can (19 oz [540 mL]) tomatoes, puréed	I
¼ cup	sliced pitted black olives	50 mL
I tsp	dried basil (or 2 tbsp [25 mL] chopped fresh)	5 mL
	Red pepper flakes	
2 oz	goat cheese	50 g
12 oz	rotini	375 g
I tbsp	grated Parmesan cheese	15 mL
	Chopped fresh parsley	

1. In large nonstick saucepan, heat oil; sauté garlic and onions for 5 minutes. Add tomatoes, olives, basil, and red pepper flakes to taste; cover and simmer for 10 minutes, stirring often. Add goat cheese, stirring until melted.

2. Meanwhile, cook pasta according to package directions or until firm to the bite. Drain and place in serving bowl. Toss with sauce. Sprinkle with Parmesan cheese and garnish with parsley.

MAKE AHEAD ◆ If serving cold, prepare and refrigerate early in day and toss again prior to serving.

PER SERVING

3	■	Starch Choices
½	◢	Fruit & Vegetable Choice
½	◲	Protein Choice
I	▲	Fat & Oil Choice

Calories 308
Carbohydrates . . . . 53 g
Fiber . . . . 4 g
Protein . . . . 11 g
Fat, total . . . . 6 g
Fat, saturated . . . . 2 g
Sodium . . . . 336 mg
Cholesterol . . . . . . 5 mg

TIP

Here's a wonderful way to use fresh salmon and not have too much protein. Fresh tuna or swordfish is a great substitute.

Fettuccine with Fresh Salmon, Dill and Leeks

4 tsp	margarine	20 mL
4 tsp	all-purpose flour	20 mL
2 cups	2% milk	500 mL
¼ cup	grated Parmesan cheese	50 mL
¼ cup	white wine	50 mL
2 tbsp	chopped onion	25 mL
1 tsp	crushed garlic	5 mL
2	leeks, washed and sliced in thin rounds	2
12 oz	fresh salmon, boned and cubed	375 g
3 tbsp	chopped fresh dill (or 1 tsp [5 mL] dried dillweed)	45 mL
10 oz	fettuccine noodles	300 g

1. In small saucepan, melt margarine; add flour and cook, stirring, for 30 seconds. Add milk and cook, stirring constantly, until thickened, 4 to 5 minutes. Stir in cheese until melted; set aside.

2. In large skillet, combine wine, onion, garlic and leeks; cook over medium heat for approximately 10 minutes or until leeks are softened. Add white sauce along with salmon. Cook for 2 to 3 minutes or until salmon is almost opaque, stirring gently. Stir in dill.

3. Meanwhile, cook fettuccine according to package directions or until firm to the bite. Drain and place in serving bowl. Toss with sauce.

MAKE AHEAD ◆ The white sauce can be prepared early in day or up to day before, but add a little extra milk when reheating before continuing with recipe.

PER SERVING

2½ ■ Starch Choices

1 �ా Fruit & Vegetable Choice

½ ◆ 2% Milk Choice

2½ ◉ Protein Choices

½ ▲ Fat & Oil Choice

Calories 410
Carbohydrates . . . . 52 g
Fiber . . . . 3 g
Protein . . . . 25 g
Fat, total . . . . 11 g
Fat, saturated . . . . 3 g
Sodium . . . . 197 mg
Cholesterol . . . . . 43 mg

Preheat oven to 350°F
(180°C)
13- by 9-inch (3 L)
baking dish

PER SERVING

| 1½ ◼ Starch Choices |
| 1 ◗ Fruit & Vegetable Choice |
| 2½ ◔ Protein Choices |
| ½ ▲ Fat & Oil Choice |

Calories 331
Carbohydrates . . . . 36 g
Fiber . . . . 2 g
Protein . . . . 22 g
Fat, total . . . . 11 g
Fat, saturated . . . . 6 g
Sodium . . . . 848 mg
Cholesterol . . . . . 90 mg

Manicotti Shells
Filled with Cheese and Smoked Salmon Bits

12	manicotti shells	12
1½ cups	ricotta cheese	375 mL
1	egg	1
2½ oz	chopped smoked salmon	60 g
¼ cup	finely chopped green onions	50 mL
3 tbsp	fresh chopped dill (or 1 tsp [5 mL] dried)	45 mL
2 tbsp	2% milk	25 mL
2 tbsp	grated Parmesan cheese	25 mL
1½ cups	prepared tomato sauce	375 mL

1. Cook pasta in boiling water according to package instructions or until firm to the bite. Drain, cover and set aside.

2. In bowl, combine ricotta cheese, egg, salmon, green onions, dill, milk and Parmesan cheese; mix until smooth. Fill pasta shells.

3. Pour half tomato sauce in bottom of large baking dish. Place pasta shells over sauce and pour other half tomato sauce over pasta. Cover and bake for 15 to 20 minutes or until hot.

MAKE AHEAD ◆ Prepare stuffed pasta shells up to a day ahead with sauce poured over. Bake just before serving.

TIPS

Ground chicken, turkey or veal can replace the beef. Chick peas can be replaced with kidney beans.

◆

Using bran flakes in the recipe also adds to the fiber content of the meal.

Spicy Meatball and Pasta Stew

MEATBALLS

8 oz	lean ground beef	250 g
1	egg	1
2 tbsp	ketchup or chili sauce	25 mL
2 tbsp	seasoned bread crumbs	25 mL
1 tsp	minced garlic	5 mL
½ tsp	chili powder	2 mL

STEW

2 tsp	vegetable oil	10 mL
1 tsp	minced garlic	5 mL
1¼ cups	chopped onions	300 mL
¾ cup	chopped carrots	175 mL
3½ cups	beef stock	875 mL
1	can (19 oz [540 mL]) tomatoes, crushed	1
¾ cup	canned chick peas, drained	175 mL
1 tbsp	tomato paste	15 mL
2 tsp	granulated sugar	10 mL
2 tsp	chili powder	10 mL
1 tsp	dried oregano	5 mL
1¼ tsp	dried basil	6 mL
⅔ cup	small shell pasta	150 mL

1. In large bowl, combine ground beef, egg, ketchup, bread crumbs, garlic and chili powder; mix well. Form each ½ tbsp (7 mL) into a meatball and place on a baking sheet; cover and set aside.

2. In large nonstick saucepan, heat oil over medium heat. Add garlic, onions and carrots and cook for 5 minutes or until onions are softened. Stir in stock, tomatoes, chick peas, tomato paste, sugar, chili powder, oregano and basil; bring to a boil, reduce heat to medium-low, cover and let cook for 20 minutes. Bring to a boil again and stir in pasta

continued on page 125

PER SERVING

½ ◼ Starch Choice

1½ ◪ Fruit & Vegetable Choices

1 ◪ Protein Choice

1 ▲ Fat & Oil Choice

Calories 203
Carbohydrates . . . . 26 g
Fiber . . . . 3 g
Protein . . . . 11 g
Fat, total . . . . 7 g
Fat, saturated . . . . 2 g
Sodium . . . . 831 mg
Cholesterol . . . . . 43 mg

and meatballs; let simmer for 10 minutes or until pasta is tender but firm, and meatballs are cooked.

MAKE AHEAD ◆ Prepare up to a day ahead, adding more stock if too thick. Great for leftovers.

❖

Turkey Macaroni Chili

Serves 8

TIPS

Great mild-tasting chili that children love. Can be served as a soup or alongside rice or pasta.

◆

Ground turkey can be replaced with ground chicken, beef or veal.

◆

Red kidney beans can be replaced with white beans or chick peas.

1½ tsp	vegetable oil	7 mL
1 tsp	minced garlic	5 mL
½ cup	finely chopped carrots	125 mL
1 cup	chopped onions	250 mL
8 oz	ground turkey	250 g
1	can (19 oz [540 mL]) tomatoes, crushed	1
2 cups	chicken stock	500 mL
1½ cups	peeled, diced potatoes	375 mL
¾ cup	canned red kidney beans, drained	175 mL
¾ cup	corn kernels	175 mL
2 tbsp	tomato paste	25 mL
1½ tsp	chili powder	7 mL
1½ tsp	dried oregano	7 mL
1½ tsp	dried basil	7 mL
⅓ cup	elbow macaroni	75 mL

1. In large nonstick saucepan, heat oil over medium heat; add garlic, carrots and onions and cook for 8 minutes or until softened, stirring occasionally. Add turkey and cook, stirring to break it up, for 2 minutes or until no longer pink. Add tomatoes, stock, potatoes, beans, corn, tomato paste, chili, oregano and basil; bring to a boil, reduce heat to low, cover and simmer for 20 minutes.

2. Bring to a boil and add macaroni; cook for 12 minutes or until pasta is tender but firm.

MAKE AHEAD ◆ Can be prepared up to 2 days ahead and reheated. Can be frozen for up to 3 weeks. Great for leftovers.

PER SERVING

1½ ■ Starch Choices

1 ◢ Fruit & Vegetable Choice

1 ◉ Protein Choice

½ ▲ Fat & Oil Choice

Calories 240
Carbohydrates . . . . 35 g
Fiber . . . . 5 g
Protein . . . . 13 g
Fat, total . . . . 6 g
Fat, saturated . . . . 0 g
Sodium . . . . 552 mg
Cholesterol . . . . . . 0 mg

Sun-Dried Tomato and Leek Pasta Bake

Serves 6 to 8

Preheat oven to 350°F (180°C)

9-inch (2.5 L) springform pan lined with foil and sprayed with vegetable spray

TIPS

To soften sun-dried tomatoes, pour boiling water over them and soak 15 minutes or until soft. Drain and chop.

◆

Any small, shaped pasta works well in this recipe. Try macaroni or orzo.

1 cup	small shell pasta	250 mL
2 tsp	vegetable oil	10 mL
2 tsp	minced garlic	10 mL
1½ cups	chopped leeks	375 mL
1½ cups	sliced mushrooms	375 mL
1 cup	chopped red bell peppers	250 mL
½ cup	chopped softened sun-dried tomatoes (see Tip, at left)	125 mL
⅓ cup	sliced black olives	75 mL
2	eggs	2
2 egg	whites	2
1 cup	2% evaporated milk	250 mL
½ cup	shredded part-skim mozzarella cheese (about 2 oz [50 g])	125 mL
2 tsp	dried basil	10 mL
3 oz	feta cheese, crumbled	75 g
2 tbsp	grated Parmesan cheese	25 mL

1. In a pot of boiling water, cook pasta 5 minutes or until tender but firm. Rinse under cold water, drain and set aside.

2. In a nonstick frying pan, heat oil over medium heat. Add garlic and leeks; cook 4 minutes or until softened. Stir in mushrooms and red peppers; cook 6 minutes or until vegetables are tender and moisture is absorbed. Stir in sun-dried tomatoes and black olives; remove from heat.

3. In a large bowl, whisk together whole eggs, egg whites, evaporated milk, mozzarella and basil. Stir in pasta, cooled vegetable mixture and feta. Pour into prepared pan. Sprinkle with Parmesan cheese.

4. Bake 30 to 35 minutes or until set.

MAKE AHEAD ◆ Prepare up to 1 day in advance. Reheat gently.

PER SERVING

½ ■ Starch Choice
1 ◧ Fruit & Vegetable Choice
½ ◆ 2% Milk Choice
1½ ◪ Protein Choices
1 ▲ Fat & Oil Choice

Calories 227
Carbohydrates . . . . 22 g
Fiber . . . . 2 g
Protein . . . . 14 g
Fat, total . . . . 10 g
Fat, saturated . . . . 5 g
Sodium . . . . 399 mg
Cholesterol . . . . . 77 mg

Serves 6

TIPS

Sauce is wonderful served over cooked vegetables, fish, chicken or meat.

◆

If prosciutto is not available, use sliced ham or smoked salmon.

Warm Caesar Pasta Salad

SAUCE

1	egg	1
3	anchovies, chopped	3
3 tbsp	olive oil	45 mL
2 tbsp	grated Parmesan cheese	25 mL
1 tbsp	lemon juice	15 mL
1 tbsp	red wine vinegar	15 mL
2 tsp	Dijon mustard	10 mL
1½ tsp	minced garlic	7 mL
2 cups	washed, dried and torn romaine lettuce	500 mL
2 oz	prosciutto, shredded	50 g
12 oz	penne	375 g

1. Put egg, anchovies, olive oil, Parmesan, lemon juice, vinegar, mustard and garlic in food processor; process until smooth.

2. Put lettuce and prosciutto in large serving bowl. In large pot of boiling water, cook pasta according to package directions or until tender but firm; drain and add to serving bowl. Pour dressing over pasta and toss.

MAKE AHEAD ◆ Prepare sauce up to a day ahead. Refrigerate. Toss just before serving.

PER SERVING

3 ■ Starch Choices

1 ◉ Protein Choice

1½ ▲ Fat & Oil Choices

Calories 344
Carbohydrates . . . . 48 g
Fiber . . . . 2 g
Protein . . . . 14 g
Fat, total . . . . 11 g
Fat, saturated . . . . 2 g
Sodium . . . . 228 mg
Cholesterol . . . . . 50 mg

PER SERVING

3	■	Starch Choices
1	◢	Fruit & Vegetable Choice
1	✱	Sugar Choice
1½	◐	Protein Choices
2	▲	Fat & Oil Choices
1	✚✚	Extra Choice

Calories 469
Carbohydrates . . . . 71 g
Fiber . . . . 4 g
Protein . . . . 17 g
Fat, total . . . . 14 g
Fat, saturated . . . . 2 g
Sodium . . . . 1171 mg
Cholesterol . . . . . 53 mg

Avocado Crab Meat over Rice Noodles

8 oz	crabmeat or surimi (imitation crab), diced	250 g
1 cup	julienned carrots	250 mL
1 cup	julienned red bell peppers	250 mL
⅓ cup	sliced green onions	75 mL
½ cup	diced ripe avocado	125 mL
¼ cup	light mayonnaise	50 mL
3 tbsp	light soya sauce	45 mL
2 tbsp	water	25 mL
2 tbsp	honey	25 mL
1 tbsp	sesame oil	15 mL
1½ tsp	minced garlic	7 mL
1½ tsp	minced gingerroot	7 mL
½ tsp	wasabi (Japanese horseradish), optional	2 mL
8 oz	wide rice noodles	250 g

1. In a serving bowl, combine crabmeat, carrots, red peppers and green onions; set aside.

2. In a food processor combine avocado, mayonnaise, soya sauce, water, honey, sesame oil, garlic, gingerroot and wasabi; process until smooth. Add to crab mixture.

3. In a large pot of boiling water, cook rice noodles for 5 minutes or until tender; drain well. Add to crab mixture; toss well. Garnish with 2 thin slices avocado. Serve immediately.

Southwest Barley Salad (page 133) ➤
Overleaf: Polenta with Chèvre, and Roasted Vegetables (page 134)

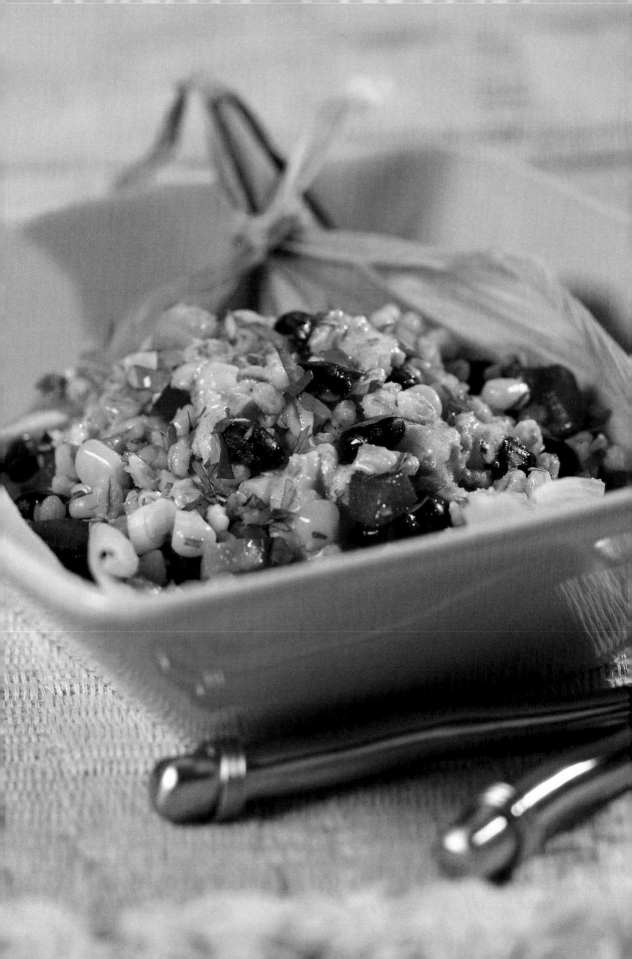

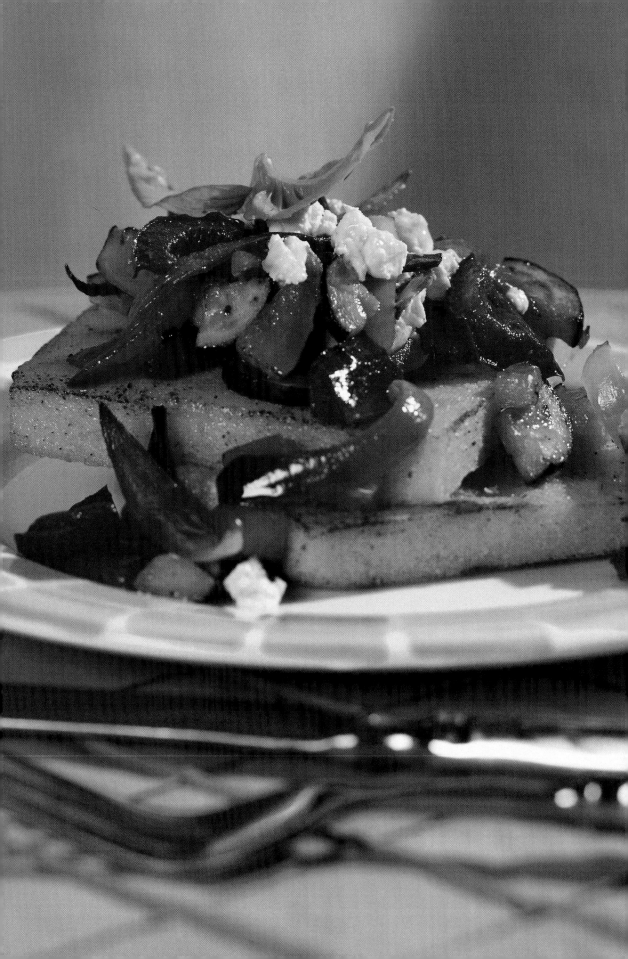

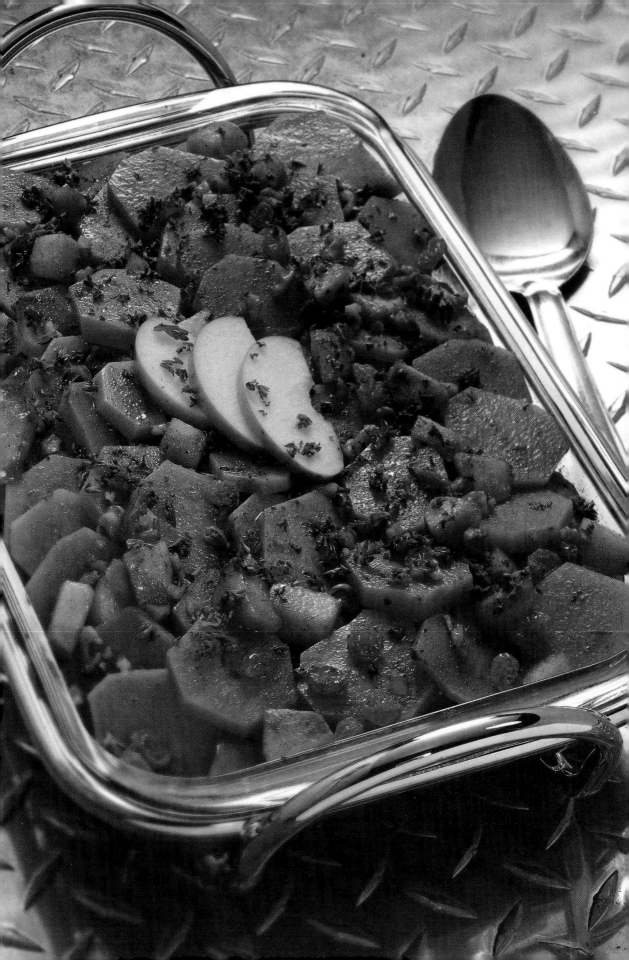

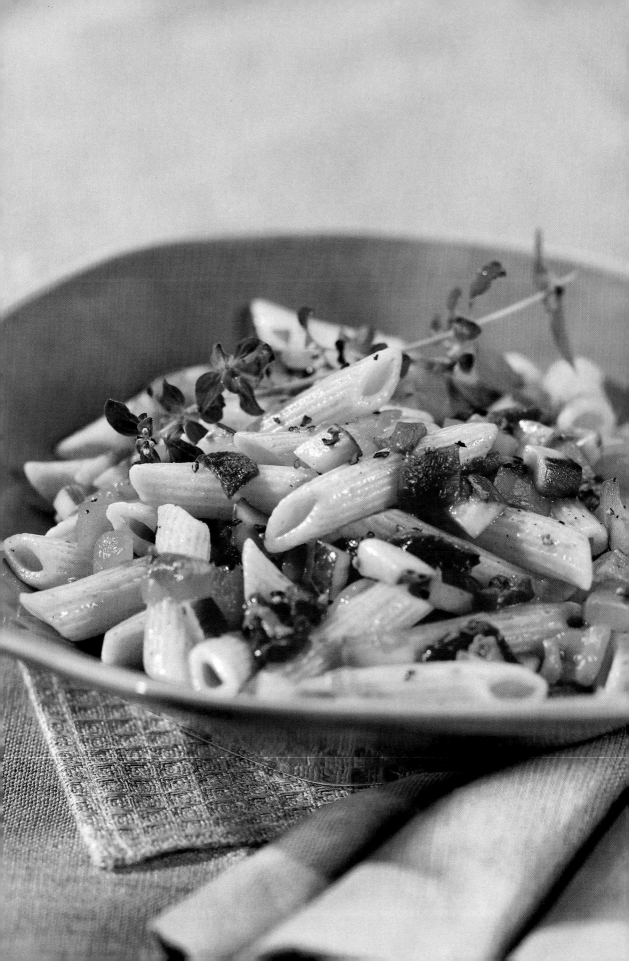

This is delicious warm or cold.

◆

Toast almonds in small skillet on top of stove or in 400°F (200°C) oven for 2 minutes.

◆

For a special dinner menu, use 1 cup (250 mL) wild rice and omit the white rice.

Wild Rice, Snow Peas and Almond Casserole

2 tsp	margarine	10 mL
½ cup	chopped onion	125 mL
1 tsp	crushed garlic	5 mL
½ cup	wild rice	125 mL
½ cup	white rice	125 mL
3¼ cups	chicken stock	800 mL
¾ cup	chopped snow peas	175 mL
¼ cup	diced sweet red pepper	50 mL
¼ cup	toasted sliced almonds	50 mL
1 tbsp	grated Parmesan cheese	15 mL

1. In large nonstick saucepan, melt margarine; sauté onion and garlic until softened. Add wild and white rice; stir for 2 minutes.

2. Add stock; reduce heat, cover and simmer just until rice is tender and liquid is absorbed, 30 to 40 minutes.

3. Add snow peas, red pepper and almonds; cook for 2 minutes. Place in serving bowl and sprinkle with cheese.

MAKE AHEAD ◆ If serving cold, prepare early in day and stir just prior to serving.

PER SERVING

2	■	Starch Choices
1	◗	Fruit & Vegetable Choice
1	◗	Protein Choice
1	▲	Fat & Oil Choice

Calories 281
Carbohydrates . . . . 42 g
Fiber . . . . 2 g
Protein . . . . 12 g
Fat, total . . . . 8 g
Fat, saturated . . . . 1 g
Sodium . . . . 654 mg
Cholesterol . . . . . . 1 mg

≺ Grilled Balsamic Vegetables over Penne (page 150)
Overleaf: Sweet Potato, Apples and Raisin Casserole (page 143)

If bok choy or nappa cabbage is unavailable, use sliced romaine or iceberg lettuce. Bok choy and nappa cabbage can be bought at Asian markets or found in the produce section of some supermarkets.

◆

Toast almonds in skillet on top of stove or in 400°F (200°C) oven for 2 minutes.

Sautéed Rice with
Almonds, Curry and Ginger

1 tbsp	vegetable oil	15 mL
1 tsp	crushed garlic	5 mL
1 ½ cups	thinly sliced bok choy or nappa cabbage	375 mL
1 cup	snow peas	250 mL
½ cup	chopped sweet red pepper	125 mL
⅓ cup	chopped carrot	75 mL
1 tsp	ground ginger	5 mL
1 tsp	curry powder	5 mL
¾ cup	chicken stock	175 mL
4 tsp	soya sauce	20 mL
1	egg	1
2 cups	cooked rice	500 mL
2 tbsp	toasted chopped almonds	25 mL
2 tbsp	chopped green onion	25 mL

1. In large nonstick skillet, heat oil; sauté garlic, cabbage, snow peas, red pepper and carrot for 3 minutes or just until tender, stirring constantly. Add ginger, curry powder, stock and soya sauce; cook for 1 minute.

2. Add egg and rice; cook for 1 minute or until egg is well incorporated. Place in serving dish and sprinkle with almonds and green onions.

MAKE AHEAD ◆ Prepare and refrigerate early in day. Just prior to serving, reheat on low heat.

PER SERVING

2	■ Starch Choices
½	▰ Fruit & Vegetable Choice
½	◙ Protein Choice
1	▲ Fat & Oil Choice
1	◆◆ Extra Choice

Calories 249
Carbohydrates . . . . 39 g
Fiber . . . . 2 g
Protein . . . . 8 g
Fat, total . . . . 7 g
Fat, saturated . . . . 1 g
Sodium . . . . 630 mg
Cholesterol . . . . . 54 mg

This dish is fine served at room temperature.

◆

Couscous is a delicious alternative to traditional ■ Starch choices. This pellet made from semolina flour is typically found in the specialty section of most supermarkets.

Couscous with Raisins, Dates and Curry

1 ¼ cups	chicken stock	300 mL
¾ cup	couscous	175 mL
1 tbsp	margarine	15 mL
¾ cup	finely chopped onions	175 mL
1 tsp	crushed garlic	5 mL
1 cup	finely chopped sweet red pepper	250 mL
¼ cup	raisins	50 mL
1 tsp	curry powder	5 mL
5	dried dates or apricots, chopped	5

1. In small saucepan, bring chicken stock to boil. Stir in couscous and remove from heat. Cover and let stand until liquid is absorbed, 5 to 8 minutes. Place in serving bowl.

2. Meanwhile, in nonstick saucepan, melt margarine; sauté onions, garlic and red pepper until softened, approximately 5 minutes. Add raisins, curry powder and dates; mix until combined. Add to couscous and mix well.

MAKE AHEAD ◆ Prepare up to the day before, then gently reheat over low heat.

PER SERVING

1½ ■ Starch Choices

2½ ◪ Fruit & Vegetable Choices

½ ▲ Fat & Oil Choice

Calories 237
Carbohydrates . . . . 49 g
Fiber . . . . 4 g
Protein . . . . 6 g
Fat, total . . . . 2 g
Fat, saturated . . . . 0 g
Sodium . . . . 480 mg
Cholesterol . . . . . . 0 mg

Although barley is rarely used this way, this dish proves how wonderful it is with tomatoes and feta cheese.

◆

Try goat cheese, instead of feta, for a change.

Barley with Sautéed Vegetables and Feta Cheese

1 tbsp	vegetable oil	15 mL
2 tsp	crushed garlic	10 mL
¾ cup	chopped sweet green pepper	175 mL
¾ cup	chopped mushrooms	175 mL
¾ cup	pot barley	175 mL
1 ½ cups	crushed canned tomatoes	375 mL
3 cups	chicken stock	750 mL
1 ½ tsp	dried basil (or 2 tbsp [25 mL] chopped fresh)	7 mL
½ tsp	dried oregano	2 mL
3 oz	feta cheese, crumbled	75 g

1. In large nonstick saucepan, heat oil; sauté garlic, green pepper and mushrooms until softened, approximately 5 minutes. Add barley and sauté for 2 minutes, stirring constantly.

2. Add tomatoes, stock, basil and oregano; cover and simmer for approximately 30 minutes or until barley is tender. Pour into serving dish and sprinkle with cheese.

MAKE AHEAD ◆ Make early in day and refrigerate; reheat on low to serve. Also delicious at room temperature.

PER SERVING

1	■	Starch Choice
1	◢	Fruit & Vegetable Choice
½	◉	Protein Choice
1	▲	Fat & Oil Choice

Calories 187
Carbohydrates . . . . 28 g
Fiber . . . . 3 g
Protein . . . . 6 g
Fat, total . . . . 6 g
Fat, saturated . . . . 3 g
Sodium . . . . 1017 mg
Cholesterol . . . . . 13 mg

Barley is one of those foods considered to be of low glycemic index. This means that there may be less rise in blood glucose after consuming this recipe in comparison to a grain of high glycemic index.

◆

A very high source of fiber, this recipe also provides an excellent source of vitamin C and riboflavin as well as good sources of phosphorus, iron, magnesium, niacin, folate and vitamins A and B$_6$.

Southwest Barley Salad

3 cups	vegetable stock (see recipe, page 46) or chicken stock	750 mL
¾ cup	pearl barley	175 mL
I cup	canned corn kernels, drained	250 mL
I cup	canned black beans, rinsed and drained	250 mL
¾ cup	chopped red bell peppers	175 mL
½ cup	chopped green bell peppers	125 mL
½ cup	chopped green onions	125 mL

DRESSING

½ cup	medium salsa	125 mL
3 tbsp	low-fat sour cream	45 mL
2 tbsp	fresh lime or lemon juice	25 mL
½ cup	chopped fresh coriander	125 mL
I tsp	minced garlic	5 mL

I. In a saucepan over high heat, bring stock to a boil. Add barley; reduce heat to medium-low. Simmer, covered, for 40 minutes or until barley is tender and liquid is absorbed. Transfer to a serving bowl; cool to room temperature. Add corn, black beans, red peppers, green peppers and green onions.

2. In a bowl combine salsa, sour cream, lime juice, coriander and garlic. Pour dressing over salad; toss to coat well.

PER SERVING

1½ ■ Starch Choices

1 ◆ Fruit & Vegetable Choice

½ ◉ Protein Choice

Calories 190
Carbohydrates . . . . 37 g
Fiber . . . . 6 g
Protein . . . . 8 g
Fat, total . . . . 2 g
Fat, saturated . . . . 1 g
Sodium . . . . 998 mg
Cholesterol . . . . . . 3 mg

Preheat oven to 425°F (220°C)

8-inch (2 L) square baking dish sprayed with vegetable spray

Large baking sheet lined with foil

TIP

Chèvre is a white, tart-flavored cheese made from goat's milk. At least, it's supposed to be — some cheese sold as chèvre contains cow's milk, so read the label carefully! Depending on the producer, goat cheese can be drier or creamier in texture. Either way, at only 15% m.f., it is a lower-fat cheese. And because it's so flavorful, a little goes a long way.

PER SERVING

1½ ■ Starch Choices

1 ● Fruit & Vegetable Choice

½ ◉ Protein Choice

1½ ▲ Fat & Oil Choices

1 ◆◆ Extra Choice

Calories 258
Carbohydrates . . . . 39 g
Fiber . . . . 4 g
Protein . . . . 9 g
Fat, total . . . . 8 g
Fat, saturated . . . . . . 3 g
Sodium . . . . 1172 mg
Cholesterol . . . . . . 7 mg

Polenta with Chèvre and Roasted Vegetables

POLENTA

3 cups	vegetable stock (see recipe, page 46) or chicken stock	750 mL
1 cup	cornmeal	250 mL
1	medium red bell pepper, cut into quarters	1
1	medium yellow pepper, cut into quarters	1
1	medium red onion, sliced	1
2	small zucchini (about 8 oz [250 g]), cut in half lengthwise	2
1 tbsp	olive oil	15 mL
1	small head garlic, top ½ inch (1 cm) cut off	1
1 tbsp	balsamic vinegar	15 mL
2 oz	goat cheese (chèvre)	50 g

1. In a deep saucepan over medium-high heat, bring stock to a boil. Reduce heat to low; gradually whisk in cornmeal. Cook, stirring, for 5 minutes. Pour into baking dish, smoothing top; chill.

2. In a bowl combine red pepper, yellow pepper, onion, zucchini and olive oil; transfer to prepared baking sheet. Wrap garlic loosely in foil; add to baking sheet. Roast vegetables in preheated oven, turning occasionally, for 45 minutes or until tender. Squeeze garlic out of skins; chop remaining vegetables. Transfer all to a bowl. Sprinkle with balsamic vinegar; toss to coat well.

3. Turn polenta onto cutting board; cut into 4 squares. In a large nonstick frying pan sprayed with vegetable spray, cook polenta over medium-high heat for 2 minutes or until golden. Turn; cook for 1 minute. Spoon polenta onto serving plates. Top with vegetable mixture; sprinkle with goat cheese. Serve.

Vegetarian Main Dishes

Many people are trying to incorporate more meatless recipes into their everyday meals. Combinations of legumes, beans, nuts and seeds and whole grains provide complete protein with less saturated fat then main courses containing animal sources of protein.

These delicious vegetarian main dishes may inspire you to venture further into the world of alternative protein choices. Canada's Food Guide recommends "incorporating dried beans, peas and lentils more often." This is a great place to start.

Flavored tortillas — such
as pesto, sun-dried
tomato, herb or whole
wheat — are now
appearing in many
supermarkets. The
different colors make
these wraps an attractive
dish for entertaining. Try
substituting other herbs
— such as coriander,
basil or parsley — for the
dill. If tahini is unavailable,
use peanut butter.

Hummus and Sautéed Vegetable Wraps

1 cup	canned chickpeas, rinsed and drained	250 mL
¼ cup	tahini	50 mL
¼ cup	water	50 mL
2 tbsp	freshly squeezed lemon juice	25 mL
4 tsp	olive oil	20 mL
1 tbsp	chopped fresh parsley	15 mL
¾ tsp	minced garlic	4 mL
2 tsp	vegetable oil	10 mL
1 cup	diced onions	250 mL
1¼ cups	diced red bell peppers	300 mL
1¼ cups	chopped snow peas	300 mL
¼ cup	chopped fresh dill (or 2 tsp [10 mL] dried)	50 mL
4	10-inch (25 cm) flour tortillas, preferably different flavors, if available	4

1. Make the hummus: In a food processor, combine chickpeas, tahini, water, lemon juice, oil, parsley and garlic; process until creamy and smooth. Transfer to a bowl and set aside.

2. In a large nonstick saucepan, heat oil over medium-high heat. Add onions and sauté 4 minutes or until soft and browned. Add red peppers and sauté 4 minutes until soft. Add snow peas and sauté 2 minutes or until tender-crisp. Stir in dill and remove from heat.

3. Divide hummus equally among tortillas, spreading to within ½ inch (1 cm) of edge. Divide vegetable mixture between tortillas. Form each tortilla into a packet by folding bottom edge over filling, then sides, then top, to enclose filling completely.

MAKE AHEAD ◆ Prepare hummus up to 3 days in advance. Sauté vegetables early in day and reheat before serving.

PER SERVING

2	■	Starch Choices
1	◆	Fruit & Vegetable Choice
1	◐	Protein Choice
3	▲	Fat & Oil Choices

Calories 382
Carbohydrates . . . . 47 g
Fiber . . . . 7 g
Protein . . . . 12 g
Fat, total . . . . 18 g
Fat, saturated . . . . 2 g
Sodium . . . . 269 mg
Cholesterol . . . . . . 0 mg

Bean Burgers
with Dill Sauce

BURGERS

2 cups	canned black beans, rinsed and drained	500 mL
½ cup	dry seasoned bread crumbs	125 mL
⅓ cup	chopped fresh dill	75 mL
⅓ cup	chopped red onions	75 mL
¼ cup	finely chopped carrots	50 mL
2 tbsp	cornmeal	25 mL
1	egg	1
1½ tsp	minced garlic	7 mL
¼ tsp	salt	1 mL

SAUCE

3 tbsp	light sour cream	45 mL
2 tbsp	light mayonnaise	25 mL
2 tsp	freshly squeezed lemon juice	10 mL
¼ to ½ tsp	minced garlic	1 to 2 mL
1 tbsp	chopped fresh dill (or ½ tsp [2 mL] dried)	15 mL

1. In a food processor, combine black beans, bread crumbs, dill, onions, carrots, cornmeal, egg, garlic and salt. Pulse on and off until well combined. With wet hands, scoop up ¼ cup (50 mL) of mixture and form into a patty. Put on prepared baking sheet. Repeat procedure for remaining patties.

2. Bake 15 minutes, turning at the halfway point.

3. Meanwhile, make the sauce: In a small bowl, stir together sour cream, mayonnaise, lemon juice, garlic and dill.

4. Serve burgers hot with sauce on side.

MAKE AHEAD ◆ Prepare mixture and sauce up to 1 day in advance. Reheat gently.

This makes an excellent total meal for vegetarians. Instead of lentils, substitute green or yellow split peas. Grilled or barbecued corn is excellent in this dish. Any type of bean can replace the red kidney beans.

◆

This is an excellent source of magnesium, phosphorus, iron, folate, zinc, vitamin C and B$_6$. With 11 g of fiber/serving, it provides about 1/3 of recommended fiber intake of 25–35 g/day.

Spicy Rice, Bean and Lentil Casserole

2 tsp	vegetable oil	10 mL
2 tsp	minced garlic	10 mL
1 cup	chopped onions	250 mL
¾ cup	chopped green peppers	175 mL
3¾ cups	basic vegetable stock (see recipe, page 46)	950 mL
¾ cup	brown rice	175 mL
½ cup	green lentils	125 mL
1 tsp	dried basil	5 mL
1 tsp	chili powder	5 mL
1	can (19 oz [540 mL]) red kidney beans, rinsed and drained	1
1 cup	canned or frozen corn kernels, drained	250 mL
1 cup	medium salsa	250 mL

1. In a nonstick saucepan, heat oil over medium-high heat. Add garlic, onions and green peppers; cook 3 minutes. Stir in stock, brown rice, lentils, basil and chili powder; bring to a boil, cover, reduce heat to medium-low and cook 30 to 40 minutes, stirring occasionally, until rice and lentils are tender and liquid is absorbed.

2. Stir in beans, corn and salsa; cover and cook 5 minutes or until heated through.

MAKE AHEAD ◆ Prepare up to 2 days in advance and reheat gently.

If using whole dried mushrooms, slice after soaking.

◆

Use any combination of wild mushrooms. If not available, use common mushrooms.

◆

The vegetables supply the majority of carbohydrate in this recipe. If this is more than the number of ✐ Fruit & Vegetable choices you usually have at one meal, count some of the carbohydrate as an extra ■ Starch choice. If you do this the recipe will be 2 ■ Starch choices and 1½ ✐ Fruit & Vegetable choices.

PER SERVING

1	■	Starch Choice
3	✐	Fruit & Vegetable Choices
½	◉	Protein Choice
½	▲	Fat & Oil Choice

Calories 252
Carbohydrates . . . . 53 g
Fiber . . . . 9 g
Protein . . . . 8 g
Fat, total . . . . 4 g
Fat, saturated . . . . 0 g
Sodium . . . . 440 mg
Cholesterol . . . . . . 0 mg

Three-Mushroom Tomato Potato Stew

1 cup	sliced dried mushrooms	250 mL
2 tsp	vegetable oil	10 mL
1½ cups	chopped onions	375 mL
2 tsp	minced garlic	10 mL
1 cup	chopped carrots	250 mL
4 cups	thinly sliced oyster mushrooms	1 L
3 cups	thinly sliced button mushrooms	750 mL
2 cups	basic vegetable stock (see recipe, page 46)	500 mL
1	can (19 oz [540 mL]) tomatoes	1
¾ cup	chopped peeled sweet potatoes	175 mL
¾ cup	chopped peeled potatoes	175 mL
2 tbsp	tomato paste	25 mL
2	bay leaves	2
1 tsp	dried basil	5 mL
1 tsp	dried thyme	5 mL
¼ tsp	coarsely ground black pepper	1 mL

1. In a small bowl, add 2 cups (500 mL) boiling water to cover dried mushrooms. Soak 15 minutes. Drain, reserving soaking liquid; measure out 1 cup (250 mL).

2. In a large nonstick saucepan sprayed with vegetable spray, heat oil over medium-high heat. Add onions, garlic and carrots; cook, stirring occasionally, 5 minutes or until softened and browned. Stir in fresh mushrooms; cook 8 minutes longer, stirring occasionally, or until all liquid is absorbed.

3. Stir in dried mushrooms, reserved 1 cup (250 mL) mushroom liquid, stock, tomatoes, sweet potatoes, potatoes, tomato paste, bay leaves, basil, thyme and pepper. Bring to a boil, reduce heat to medium-low, cover, and cook 20 minutes or until potatoes are tender.

MAKE AHEAD ◆ Prepare up to 1 day in advance. Reheat gently, adding more stock if too thick.

Replace coriander with dill or parsley.

◆

Peanut butter can replace tahini.

◆

These burgers are an excellent meatless main dish. The tahini is the source of most of the fat in this recipe. Like other nuts and seeds, the fat is primarily from monounsaturated sources.

Falafel Burgers
with Creamy Sesame Sauce

2 cups	drained canned chick peas	500 mL
1/4 cup	chopped green onions	50 mL
1/4 cup	chopped fresh coriander	50 mL
1/4 cup	finely chopped carrots	50 mL
1/4 cup	bread crumbs	50 mL
3 tbsp	lemon juice	45 mL
3 tbsp	water	45 mL
2 tbsp	tahini (puréed sesame seeds)	25 mL
2 tsp	minced garlic	10 mL
1/4 tsp	ground black pepper	1 mL
2 tsp	vegetable oil	10 mL

SAUCE

1/4 cup	light sour cream	50 mL
2 tbsp	tahini	25 mL
2 tbsp	chopped fresh coriander	25 mL
2 tbsp	water	25 mL
2 tsp	lemon juice	10 mL
1/2 tsp	minced garlic	2 mL

1. Put chick peas, green onions, coriander, carrots, bread crumbs, lemon juice, water, tahini, garlic and black pepper in food processor; pulse on and off until finely chopped. With wet hands, form each 1/4 cup (50 mL) into a patty.

2. In small bowl, whisk together sour cream, tahini, coriander, water, lemon juice and garlic.

3. In nonstick skillet sprayed with vegetable spray, heat 1 tsp (5 mL) of oil over medium heat. Add 4 patties and cook for 3 1/2 minutes or until golden; turn and cook 3 1/2 minutes longer or until golden and hot inside. Remove from pan. Heat remaining 1 tsp (5 mL) oil and cook remaining patties. Serve with sesame sauce.

MAKE AHEAD ◆ Prepare burgers early in the day and refrigerate until ready to cook. Prepare sauce to up a day ahead.

PER SERVING

1 1/2	◼	Starch Choices
1/2	◢	Fruit & Vegetable Choice
1	◉	Protein Choice
2	▲	Fat & Oil Choices
1	✦✦	Extra Choice

Calories 305
Carbohydrates . . . . 36 g
Fiber . . . . 6 g
Protein . . . . 12 g
Fat, total . . . . 14 g
Fat, saturated . . . . 3 g
Sodium . . . . 87 mg
Cholesterol . . . . . . 6 mg

Vegetables

Vegetables come in all shapes, sizes and flavors. When meal planning for diabetes, they are often grouped by their carbohydrate content. Using the Good Health Eating Guide system of meal planning you will find vegetables in three groups, potatoes and corn as part of ▣ Starch choices, many as ◗ Fruit & Vegetable choices and the low-carbohydrate ones as part of the ⊹ Extras.

Most are great sources of nutrients and many contain the phytochemicals which have been linked to potential protective effects against cancer, heart disease, osteoporosis and diabetes.

Here are some delicious ways to incorporate vegetables into your meal plan.

TIPS

The potatoes can also
be diced.

◆

Substitute another
cheese of your choice,
such as Swiss or
mozzarella.

◆

The milk and cheese in
this casserole make it
an excellent source of
calcium. Using low fat
cheese can reduce the
fat content in this
recipe to 7 g or 1 ▲
Fat & Oil Choice.

PER SERVING

1½ ■ Starch Choices

½ ◆ 2% Milk Choice

1 ⊘ Protein Choice

1½ ▲ Fat & Oil Choices

Calories 252
Carbohydrates . . . . 27 g
Fiber . . . . 2 g
Protein . . . . 12 g
Fat, total . . . . 11 g
Fat, saturated . . . . 7 g
Sodium . . . . 263 mg
Cholesterol . . . . . 32 mg

Potato Cheese Casserole

4	medium potatoes, peeled and thinly sliced	4
1½ tsp	margarine	7 mL
1 cup	chopped onions	250 mL
1 tsp	crushed garlic	5 mL
2 tbsp	all-purpose flour	25 mL
1¾ cups	2% warm milk	425 mL
3 tbsp	chopped fresh dill (or 1 tsp [5 mL] dried dillweed) Salt and pepper	45 mL
½ cup	shredded Cheddar cheese	125 mL

1. In saucepan of boiling water, cook potatoes just until fork-tender, approximately 10 minutes; drain. Arrange in baking dish just large enough to lay in single layer of overlapping slices.

2. In medium nonstick saucepan, melt margarine; sauté onions and garlic for 5 minutes or until softened. Add flour and cook, stirring, for 1 minute. Slowly stir in milk, simmer until thickened, stirring constantly, 3 to 4 minutes. Add dill; season with salt and pepper to taste.

3. Pour sauce over potatoes; sprinkle with cheese. Cover and bake for approximately 1 hour or until potatoes are tender.

MAKE AHEAD ◆ This casserole can be prepared and refrigerated up to 24 hours ahead of time and baked just prior to eating.

Preheat oven to 350°F
(180°C)

Baking dish sprayed
with nonstick
vegetable spray

The darker the skin of
the sweet potato, the
moister it is.

◆

This recipe should be
reserved for special
occasions as it is relatively
high in carbohydrate for
an everyday meal. The
honey or maple syrup
can be replaced with
granulated sugar sub-
stitute to save about 14 g
of carbohydrate/serving
and eliminate the
1½ ✴ Sugars choices.

◆

Chopped dates or
apricots can replace
the raisins.

PER SERVING

1	◼	Starch Choice
1	◢	Fruit & Vegetable Choice
1½	✴	Sugar Choices
1	▲	Fat & Oil Choice

Calories 216
Carbohydrates . . . . 42 g
Fiber . . . . 3 g
Protein . . . . 2 g
Fat, total . . . . 6 g
Fat, saturated . . . . 1 g
Sodium . . . . 60 mg
Cholesterol . . . . . . 0 mg

Sweet Potato, Apple and Raisin Casserole

1 lb	sweet potatoes, peeled and cubed	500 g
¾ tsp	ground ginger	4 mL
¼ cup	honey or maple syrup	50 mL
¾ tsp	ground cinnamon	4 mL
2 tbsp	margarine, melted	25 mL
¼ cup	raisins	50 mL
2 tbsp	chopped walnuts	25 mL
¾ cup	cubed peeled sweet apples	175 mL

1. Steam or microwave sweet potatoes just until slightly underdone. Drain and place in baking dish.

2. In small bowl, combine ginger, honey, cinnamon, margarine, raisins, walnuts and apples; mix well. Pour over sweet potatoes and bake, uncovered, for 20 minutes or until tender.

MAKE AHEAD ◆ Prepare casserole without apples up to the day before. Add apples, toss and bake just prior to serving.

Serves 4

Adjust the lemon to taste.

◆

If asparagus is not available, try broccoli.

◆

This recipe is a good source of folate and vitamin C. A delicious accompaniment to a meal.

Asparagus with Lemon and Garlic

½ lb	asparagus, trimmed	250 g
2 tsp	vegetable oil	10 mL
1 tsp	crushed garlic	5 mL
¼ cup	diced sweet red pepper	50 mL
1	green onion, sliced	1
2 tbsp	white wine	25 mL
4 tsp	lemon juice	20 mL
2 tbsp	chicken stock	25 mL
	Pepper	

1. Steam or boil asparagus just until tender-crisp. Do not overcook. Drain and set aside.

2. In large nonstick skillet, heat oil; sauté garlic and red pepper until softened.

3. Reduce heat and add green onion, wine, lemon juice, chicken stock, pepper to taste and asparagus. Cook for 1 minute. Place asparagus mixture in serving dish.

MAKE AHEAD ◆ Make this early in day if it is to be served cold, to allow the asparagus a chance to marinate.

PER SERVING

½ ▲ Fat & Oil Choice

1 ◆◆ Extra Choice

Calories	39
Carbohydrates	3 g
Fiber	1 g
Protein	1 g
Fat, total	2 g
Fat, saturated	0 g
Sodium	46 mg
Cholesterol	0 mg

Brussels sprouts can have a slightly bitter taste, especially if overcooked. The addition of sweet potatoes and pecans balances the flavor.

◆

Toast pecans in 400°F (200°C) oven or in skillet on top of stove for 2 minutes or until brown.

◆

With relatively little change in taste, the brown sugar or honey can be replaced with granulated sugar substitute to save about 5 g of carbohydrate/serving and eliminate the ½ ✱ Sugar choice.

PER SERVING

1	■	Starch Choice
½	▰	Fruit & Vegetable Choice
½	✱	Sugar Choice
½	◉	Protein Choice
1	▲	Fat & Oil Choice

Calories 186
Carbohydrates . . . . 32 g
Fiber . . . . 6 g
Protein . . . . 6 g
Fat, total . . . . 6 g
Fat, saturated . . . . . . 1 g
Sodium . . . . 152 mg
Cholesterol . . . . . . 0 mg

Brussels Sprouts with
Pecans and Sweet Potatoes

1½ cups	cubed peeled sweet potatoes	375 mL
¾ lb	brussels sprouts, cut in half	375 g
1 tbsp	margarine	15 mL
½ cup	chopped onion	125 mL
1 tsp	crushed garlic	5 mL
¼ cup	chicken stock	50 mL
4 tsp	brown sugar or honey	20 mL
¼ tsp	cinnamon	1 mL
2 tbsp	pecan pieces, toasted	25 mL

1. In saucepan of boiling water, cook sweet potatoes until just tender; drain and reserve. Repeat with brussels sprouts. Set aside.

2. In nonstick skillet, melt margarine; sauté onion and garlic just until tender. Add sweet potatoes, brussels sprouts, stock, sugar, cinnamon and pecans; cook for 3 minutes or until vegetables are tender.

Add a sprinkle of fresh herbs such as parsley or basil to oil mixture.

◆

An excellent source of vitamin C.

Green Beans and Diced Tomatoes

8 oz	green beans, trimmed	250 g
1 ½ tsp	vegetable oil	7 mL
1 tsp	crushed garlic	5 mL
¾ cup	chopped onion	175 mL
⅓ cup	chopped sweet red or yellow pepper	75 mL
1 ½ cups	diced tomatoes	375 mL
½ tsp	dried basil (or 1 tbsp [15 mL] fresh)	2 mL
½ tsp	dried oregano	2 mL
2 tbsp	chicken stock	25 mL
2 tsp	lemon juice	10 mL
2 tsp	grated Parmesan cheese (optional)	10 mL

1. Steam or microwave green beans just until tender. Set aside.

2. In nonstick skillet, heat oil; sauté garlic, onion and red pepper just until tender.

3. Add green beans, tomatoes, basil, oregano, stock and lemon juice; cook for 2 minutes, stirring constantly. Serve sprinkled with Parmesan (if using).

MAKE AHEAD ◆ These peppers can be prepared ahead of time and served cold.

PER SERVING

| 1 | ◢ Fruit & Vegetable Choice |
| ½ | ▲ Fat & Oil Choice |

Calories. 77
Carbohydrates . . . . 13 g
Fiber . . . . 3 g
Protein . . . . 3 g
Fat, total . . . . 3 g
Fat, saturated . . . . 0 g
Sodium . . . . 74 mg
Cholesterol . . . . . . 1 mg

Preheat oven to 400°F (200°C)

Add a sprinkle of fresh herbs such as parsley or basil to oil mixture.

◆

This is a delicious and colorful way to serve sweet peppers. When eaten in quantity some ⧉ Extra vegetables become ◪ Fruit & Vegetable choices.

Roasted Garlic Sweet Pepper Strips

4	large sweet peppers (combination of green, red and yellow)	4
2 tbsp	olive oil	25 mL
1½ tsp	crushed garlic	7 mL
1 tbsp	grated Parmesan cheese	15 mL

1. On baking sheet, bake whole peppers for 15 to 20 minutes, turning occasionally, or until blistered and blackened. Place in paper bag; seal and let stand for 10 minutes.

2. Peel off charred skin from peppers; cut off tops and bottoms. Remove seeds and ribs; cut into 1 inch (2.5 cm) wide strips and place on serving platter.

3. Mix oil with garlic; brush over peppers. Sprinkle with cheese.

MAKE AHEAD ◆ These peppers can be prepared ahead of time and served cold.

PER SERVING

1	◪ Fruit & Vegetable Choice
1½ ▲ Fat & Oil Choices	

Calories	112
Carbohydrates	11 g
Fiber	2 g
Protein	2 g
Fat, total	8 g
Fat, saturated	1 g
Sodium	30 mg
Cholesterol	1 mg

TIPS

Use any other combination of vegetables. Keep colors contrasting.

◆

A delicious combination of vegetables serving as an excellent source of vitamins A and C. Serve with traditional meals to brighten up any ordinary supper.

◆

Remember to cook on a high heat and not to overcook.

Teriyaki Sesame Vegetables

1½ tsp	vegetable oil	7 mL
1 tsp	crushed garlic	5 mL
Half	large sweet red or yellow pepper, sliced thinly	Half
Half	large sweet green pepper, sliced thinly	Half
1½ cups	snow peas	375 mL
1	large carrot, sliced thinly	1
½ tsp	sesame seeds	2 mL

SAUCE

1 tsp	crushed garlic	5 mL
1 tbsp	soya sauce	15 mL
1 tbsp	rice wine vinegar or white wine vinegar	15 mL
½ tsp	minced gingerroot	2 mL
½ tsp	sesame oil	2 mL
1 tbsp	water	15 mL
1 tbsp	brown sugar	15 mL
1½ tsp	vegetable oil	7 mL

1. Sauce: In small saucepan, combine garlic, soya sauce, vinegar, ginger, sesame oil, water, sugar and vegetable oil; cook for 3 to 5 minutes or until thickened and syrupy.

2. In large nonstick skillet, heat oil; sauté garlic, red and green peppers, snow peas and carrot, stirring constantly, for 2 minutes.

3. Add sauce; sauté for 2 minutes or just until vegetables are tender-crisp. Place in serving dish and sprinkle with sesame seeds.

The texture and flavor of wild mushrooms warrants the expense. If they are unavailable, use regular mushrooms.

◆

Try plum tomatoes instead of field tomatoes.

◆

This vegetable dish is almost a meal in itself. Prepare a custard for dessert, which could use a granulated sugar substitute. The meal will be complete with the added ◪ Protein and ◆ Milk choices found in the custard.

PER SERVING

3	■	Starch Choices
1	◪	Fruit & Vegetable Choice
½	◆	2% Milk Choice
½	◪	Protein Choice
½	▲	Fat & Oil Choice

Calories 346
Carbohydrates . . . . 62 g
Fiber . . . . 4 g
Protein . . . . 13 g
Fat, total . . . . 5 g
Fat, saturated . . . . 2 g
Sodium . . . . 63 mg
Cholesterol . . . . . . 6 mg

Penne with Wild Mushrooms

12 oz	penne	375 g
1 tsp	margarine or butter	5 mL
3 cups	sliced wild mushrooms (oyster, cremini, portobello)	750 mL
2 tsp	olive oil	10 mL
2 tsp	crushed garlic	10 mL
1 cup	diced onions	250 mL
1 lb	chopped tomatoes (about 3 cups [750 mL])	500 g
2 cups	2% milk	500 mL
4 tsp	all-purpose flour	20 mL
½ cup	fresh chopped basil (or 2 tsp [10 mL] dried) Pepper	125 mL

1. Cook pasta in boiling water according to package instructions or until firm to the bite. Drain and place in serving bowl.

2. In large nonstick skillet, melt margarine; sauté mushrooms for 5 minutes. Drain off excess liquid. Add oil; sauté garlic and onions just until tender, approximately 3 minutes. Add tomatoes; simmer on low heat for 10 minutes just until tomatoes become very soft.

3. Meanwhile, in small bowl, mix milk and flour until smooth; add to tomato mixture and simmer on medium heat for 3 minutes or until sauce thickens slightly. Pour over pasta. Sprinkle with basil and pepper, and toss.

MAKE AHEAD ◆ Prepare sauce early in day, leaving at room temperature. Reheat gently, adding more milk if too thick.

Preheat oven to broil or start barbecue

Grilled Balsamic Vegetables over Penne

1	medium red onion, cut in half horizontally	1
1	medium zucchini, cut lengthwise into 4 strips	1
3	medium sweet peppers (green, red and/or yellow)	3
2	medium tomatoes, cut in half horizontally	2
1 lb	penne	500 g

DRESSING

3 tbsp	lemon juice	45 mL
3 tbsp	balsamic vinegar	45 mL
¼ cup	olive oil	50 mL
2 tsp	crushed garlic	10 mL

1. Place all vegetables on grill or barbecue. Grill onion for 25 minutes, turning until charred. Grill zucchini for 15 minutes until charred, turning as necessary. Grill sweet peppers for 15 minutes until charred. Grill tomatoes for 12 to 15 minutes until charred, rotating as necessary. Let vegetables cool for 10 minutes.

2. Remove top, skin and seeds of sweet peppers. Chop all vegetables into medium diced pieces, keeping juices. Set aside.

3. Meanwhile, cook pasta in boiling water according to package instructions or until firm to the bite. Drain and place in serving bowl. Add vegetables.

4. Make the dressing: Combine lemon juice, vinegar, oil and garlic. Pour over pasta, and toss.

MAKE AHEAD ◆ Grill vegetables early in day. Chop before cooking pasta.

PER SERVING

3	■	Starch Choices
1	◢	Fruit & Vegetable Choice
1½	▲	Fat & Oil Choices

Calories 324
Carbohydrates . . . . 54 g
Fiber . . . . 4 g
Protein . . . . 9 g
Fat, total . . . . 9 g
Fat, saturated . . . . 1 g
Sodium . . . . 9 mg
Cholesterol . . . . . . 0 mg

Preheat oven to 425°F
(220°C)

Baking sheet sprayed
with vegetable spray

These mushrooms can
serve as a wonderful
appetizer or side dish
with a main meal.

◆

Use fresh parsley or
spinach to replace basil,
or use a combination.
Toast pine nuts in a
nonstick skillet for
2 minutes until browned.

Cheesy Pesto Stuffed Mushrooms

14 oz	large stuffing mushrooms (approximately 16)	350 g
¾ cup	packed basil leaves	175 mL
1 ½ tbsp	olive oil	20 mL
1 ½ tbsp	toasted pine nuts	20 mL
1 tbsp	grated Parmesan cheese	15 mL
½ tsp	minced garlic	2 mL
2 tbsp	chicken stock or water	25 mL
¼ cup	5% ricotta cheese	50 mL

1. Wipe mushrooms clean and gently remove stems; reserve for another purpose. Put caps on baking sheet.

2. Put basil, olive oil, pine nuts, Parmesan and garlic in food processor; process until finely chopped, scraping down sides of bowl once. Add stock through the feed tube and process until smooth. Add ricotta and process until mixed.

3. Divide mixture evenly among mushroom caps. Bake for 10 to 15 minutes or until hot.

MAKE AHEAD ◆ Prepare filling up to a day ahead. Fill mushrooms early in the day. Bake just before serving.

PER SERVING

½ ◢ Fruit & Vegetable Choice

½ ◢ Protein Choice

½ ▲ Fat & Oil Choice

Calories 68
Carbohydrates . . . . . 4 g
Fiber . . . . 1 g
Protein . . . . 3 g
Fat, total . . . . 5 g
Fat, saturated . . . . 1 g
Sodium . . . . 62 mg
Cholesterol . . . . . . 4 mg

Baked Potatoes
Stuffed with Smoked Salmon and Broccoli

4	medium baking potatoes	4
1 cup	chopped broccoli florets	250 mL
2/3 cup	light sour cream	150 mL
1/4 cup	2% milk	50 mL
1/4 cup	grated Parmesan cheese	50 mL
2 tbsp	chopped fresh dill (or 2 tsp [10 mL] dried)	25 mL
1/4 cup	chopped green onions (about 2 medium)	50 mL
3 oz	smoked salmon, chopped	75 g

1. Bake the potatoes for 1 hour or until easily pierced with a fork; let cool slightly. Meanwhile, in a saucepan of boiling water or in microwave, cook the broccoli for 1 minute or until tender-crisp. Drain and set aside.

2. Cut potatoes in half lengthwise, and carefully scoop out flesh, leaving skins intact. Mash potato with sour cream and milk; stir in 2 tbsp (25 mL) of the Parmesan, the dill, green onions, smoked salmon and broccoli. Spoon mixture back into potato skin shells; sprinkle with remaining 2 tbsp (25 mL) Parmesan. Bake for 10 to 15 minutes, or until heated through.

MAKE AHEAD ◆ Prepare filling up to a day ahead and fill potatoes. Bake just before serving.

Serves 6

Preheat oven to 350°F (180°C)

2-quart (2 L) casserole dish sprayed with vegetable spray

TIPS

Be sure to use evaporated milk — it's what gives this dish its creaminess.

◆

Leeks can have a lot of hidden dirt — to clean thoroughly, slice in half lengthwise and wash under cold running water, getting between the layers where dirt hides.

◆

Use fresh parsley, basil or coriander instead of dill. Reheat leftovers gently.

PER SERVING

I	Starch Choice	
½	◗ Fruit & Vegetable Choice	
½	◆ 2% Milk Choice	
½	Protein Choice	

Calories 169
Carbohydrates . . . . 26 g
Fiber . . . . 2 g
Protein . . . . 8 g
Fat, total . . . . 5 g
Fat, saturated . . . . I g
Sodium . . . . 110 mg
Cholesterol . . . . . 76 mg

Corn, Leek and Red Pepper Casserole

I tsp	vegetable oil	5 mL
I tsp	minced garlic	5 mL
I cup	sliced leeks	250 mL
I cup	chopped red peppers	250 mL
2 cups	corn kernels	500 mL
2½ tbsp	all-purpose flour	35 mL
2	whole eggs	2
2	egg whites	2
1⅓ cups	2% evaporated milk	325 mL
¼ cup	chopped fresh dill (or 2 tsp [10 mL] dried)	50 mL
¼ cup	bread crumbs	50 mL
½ tsp	margarine or butter	2 mL

1. In nonstick skillet sprayed with vegetable spray, heat oil over medium heat. Add garlic, leeks and red peppers and cook for 7 minutes, or until tender, stirring occasionally; set aside.

2. Put 1 cup (250 mL) of corn in food processor with flour; purée. Add whole eggs, egg whites, evaporated milk and dill; process until smooth.

3. In large bowl, combine sautéed vegetables, corn purée and remaining 1 cup (250 mL) corn. Pour into prepared dish. Combine bread crumbs and margarine until crumbly. Sprinkle over top casserole and bake for 30 minutes or until set at center.

MAKE AHEAD ◆ Cook vegetables early in day. Bake dish just before serving.

Preheat oven to 350°F
(180°C)

8-inch (2 L) springform
pan sprayed with
vegetable spray

TIPS

Use a 10-oz (300 g)
package of frozen
spinach instead of fresh
spinach. All ricotta or all
cottage cheese can be
used, but ricotta gives a
creamy texture.

◆

Serve this quiche with
fresh whole grain bread.
Half a cup (125 mL)
of no sugar added
raspberry yogurt
served over 1 cup
(250 mL) of fresh
raspberries or a sliced
peach make the
meal complete.

PER SERVING

½ ✔ Fruit & Vegetable
Choice

2 ✔ Protein Choices

1 ▲ Fat & Oil Choice

Calories 177
Carbohydrates . . . . . 7 g
Fiber . . . . 2 g
Protein . . . . 14 g
Fat, total . . . . 10 g
Fat, saturated . . . . . . 5 g
Sodium . . . . 302 mg
Cholesterol . . . . . 62 mg

Crustless Dill Spinach Quiche
with Mushrooms and Cheese

10 oz	fresh spinach	300 g
2 tsp	vegetable oil	10 mL
1 tsp	minced garlic	5 mL
¾ cup	chopped onions	175 mL
¾ cup	chopped mushrooms	175 mL
⅔ cup	5% ricotta cheese	150 mL
⅔ cup	2% cottage cheese	150 mL
⅓ cup	grated Cheddar cheese	75 mL
2 tbsp	grated Parmesan cheese	25 mL
1	whole egg	1
1	egg white	1
3 tbsp	chopped fresh dill (or 2 tsp [10 mL] dried)	45 mL
¼ tsp	ground black pepper	1 mL

1. Wash spinach and shake off excess water. In the water clinging to the leaves, cook the spinach over high heat just until it wilts. Squeeze out excess moisture, chop and set aside.

2. In large nonstick skillet, heat oil over medium heat; add garlic, onions and mushrooms and cook for 5 minutes or until softened. Remove from heat and add chopped spinach, ricotta, cottage, Cheddar and Parmesan cheeses, whole egg, egg white, dill and pepper; mix well. Pour into prepared pan and bake for 35 to 40 minutes or until knife inserted in center comes out clean.

MAKE AHEAD ◆ Prepare mixture early in the day. Bake just before serving. Great reheated gently the next day.

Sauces, Marinades and Dressings

Many commercial sauces, marinades and dressings can wreak havoc on your attempts to control your fat and carbohydrate intake. When shopping for these, read the labels carefully, keeping in mind that 5 g of fat is the equivalent of 1 teaspoon (5 mL) oil and 4 g of carbohydrate is the same as 1 teaspoon (5mL) sugar.

In most of these commercial products if one nutrient is reduced the other is increased. Try some of these homemade favorites. In those where there is "added sugar", using a granulated sugar substitute of your choice can reduce the carbohydrate content and usually eliminate the ✳ Sugars Choice.

❖

TIP

Serve over a variety of mild-tasting lettuce leaves (Boston, red, leafy).

Herb Vinaigrette

1 tbsp	red wine vinegar	15 mL
4 tsp	water	20 mL
4 tsp	lemon juice	20 mL
½ tsp	Dijon mustard	2 mL
¾ tsp	crushed garlic	4 mL
2 tbsp	chopped fresh basil (or ½ tsp [2 mL] dried)	25 mL
	Salt and pepper	
2 tbsp	vegetable oil	25 mL

1. In small bowl, whisk together vinegar, water, lemon juice, mustard, garlic, basil, and salt and pepper to taste; whisk in oil until combined.

MAKE AHEAD ◆ Refrigerate for up to 3 weeks.

PER SERVING

1   ▲ Fat & Oil Choice

Calories 51	
Carbohydrates . . . . . 1 g	
Fiber . . . . 0 g	
Protein . . . . 0 g	
Fat, total . . . . 6 g	
Fat, saturated . . . . 0 g	
Sodium . . . . 289 mg	
Cholesterol . . . . . . 0 mg	

Makes 1 cup (250 mL)

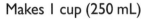
TIP

Use in a seafood salad,
or serve as a tartar
sauce with grilled fish.

Light Creamy
Dill Dressing

½ cup	2% yogurt	125 mL
2 tbsp	light mayonnaise	25 mL
3 tbsp	chopped fresh parsley	45 mL
¼ cup	chopped fresh dill (or 1½ tsp [7 mL] dried dillweed)	50 mL
1 tsp	Dijon mustard	5 mL
¾ tsp	crushed garlic	4 mL
	Salt and pepper	

1. In bowl, combine yogurt, mayonnaise, parsley, dill, mustard, garlic, and salt and pepper to taste until well mixed.

MAKE AHEAD ◆ Refrigerate for up to 1 day.

PER SERVING

1 ✦✦ Extra Choice

Calories 11
Carbohydrates . . . . . 1 g
Fiber . . . . 0 g
Protein . . . . 0 g
Fat, total . . . . 1 g
Fat, saturated . . . . 0 g
Sodium . . . . 36 mg
Cholesterol . . . . . . 1 mg

Great over leafy lettuce or spinach.

◆

For a stronger orange flavor, add 1 tsp (5 mL) grated orange zest.

◆

Balsamic vinegar is commonly found in the specialty section most supermarkets and it contributes to a wonderful flavor wherever it is added.

Balsamic Orange Vinaigrette

¼ cup	chopped fresh parsley	50 mL
3 tbsp	vegetable oil	45 mL
3 tbsp	balsamic vinegar	45 mL
3 tbsp	minced red onions	45 mL
2 tbsp	orange juice concentrate	25 mL
1 tbsp	packed brown sugar	15 mL
1 tsp	minced garlic	5 mL

1. In a small bowl, whisk together parsley, oil, vinegar, red onions, orange juice concentrate, sugar and garlic.

MAKE AHEAD ◆ Prepare up to 2 days in advance.

PER SERVING

| ½ | 🍃 Fruit & Vegetable Choice |
| 1 | ▲ Fat & Oil Choice |

| Calories . . . . 50 |
| Carbohydrates . . . . . 4 g |
| Fiber . . . . 0 g |
| Protein . . . . 0 g |
| Fat, total . . . . 4 g |
| Fat, saturated . . . . 0 g |
| Sodium . . . . 2 mg |
| Cholesterol . . . . . . 0 mg |

Serve as a dipping sauce for fruit spears or serve over a salad of spinach, orange slices and red onions.

◆

This is a great recipe for those who like sweet dressings rather than tart.

Creamy Poppy Seed Dressing

¼ cup	orange juice	50 mL
3 tbsp	light mayonnaise	45 mL
3 tbsp	light sour cream	45 mL
1 tbsp	honey	15 mL
2 tsp	poppy seeds	10 mL
1 tsp	grated orange zest	5 mL

1. In a small bowl, whisk together orange juice, mayonnaise, sour cream, honey, poppy seeds and orange zest.

MAKE AHEAD ◆ Prepare up to 2 days in advance.

PER SERVING

½ ✳ Sugar Choice

½ ▲ Fat & Oil Choice

Calories 28
Carbohydrates . . . . . 3 g
Fiber . . . . 0 g
Protein . . . . 0 g
Fat, total . . . . 2 g
Fat, saturated . . . . 0 g
Sodium . . . . 22 mg
Cholesterol . . . . . . 2 mg

Makes ½ cup (125 ml)

TIP

Serve over salad, stir-fried vegetables or rice noodles. Also great over steamed vegetables.

Thai Lime Dressing

3 tbsp	chopped fresh coriander	45 mL
2 tbsp	vegetable oil	25 mL
2 tbsp	freshly squeezed lime juice	25 mL
2 tbsp	peanut butter	25 mL
1 tbsp	rice wine vinegar	15 mL
1 tbsp	packed brown sugar	15 mL
1 tsp	sesame oil	5 mL
½ tsp	minced garlic	2 mL
½ tsp	minced gingerroot	2 mL
1	green onion, chopped	1

1. In a food processor combine coriander, oil, lime juice, peanut butter, vinegar, brown sugar, sesame oil, garlic, ginger and green onion; process until smooth.

MAKE AHEAD ◆ Prepare up to 3 days in advance. Stir before using.

PER SERVING

½ ✳ Sugar Choice

1 ▲ Fat & Oil Choice

Calories 68
Carbohydrates . . . . . 3 g
Fiber . . . . 0 g
Protein . . . . 1 g
Fat, total . . . . 6 g
Fat, saturated . . . . 1 g
Sodium . . . . 3 mg
Cholesterol . . . . . . 0 mg

Lemon Poppy Seed Loaf (page 166) ➤

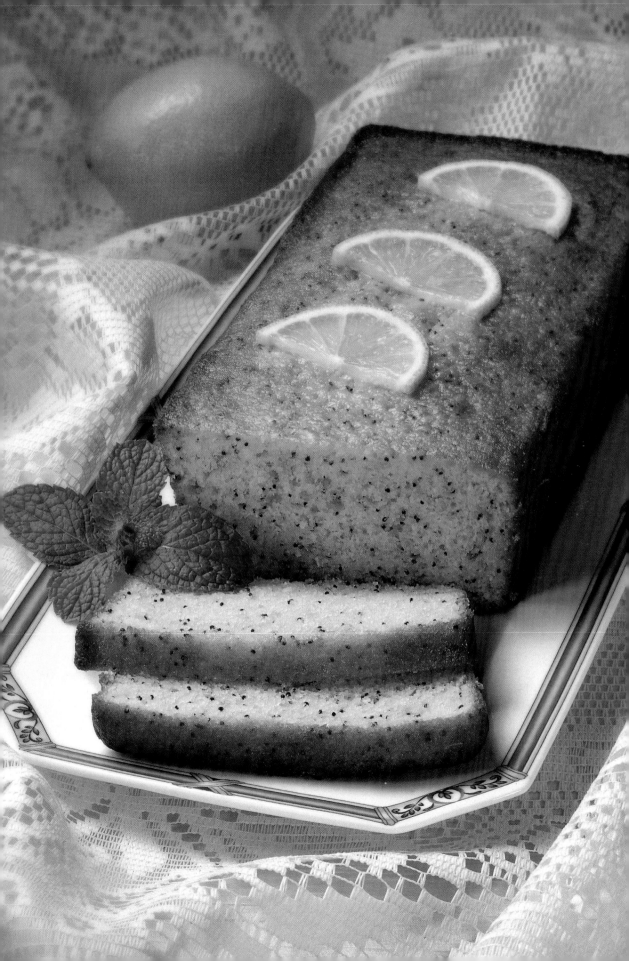

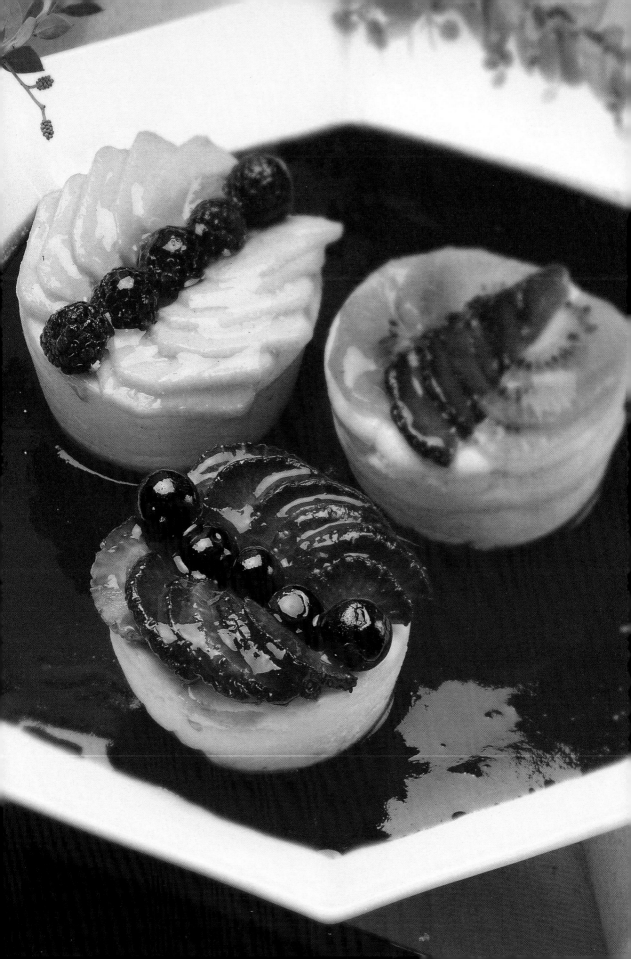

Use to marinate chicken, fish or veal. Remove meat and boil marinade for 3 to 5 minutes until thickened. Brush over meat before cooking.

◆

A granulated sugar substitute can replace the brown sugar in this recipe to eliminate the [✴] Sugars Choice.

Ginger Lemon Marinade

3 tbsp	lemon juice	45 mL
2 tbsp	water	25 mL
1 tbsp	vegetable oil	15 mL
1½ tsp	red wine vinegar	7 mL
4 tsp	brown sugar	20 mL
2 tsp	sesame oil	10 mL
1 tsp	minced gingerroot (or ¼ tsp [1 mL] ground ginger)	5 mL
½ tsp	ground coriander	2 mL
½ tsp	ground fennel seeds (optional)	2 mL

1. In small bowl, combine lemon juice, water, vegetable oil, vinegar, sugar, sesame oil, ginger, coriander, and fennel seeds (if using); mix well.

MAKE AHEAD ◆ Prepare up to 2 days in advance and refrigerate.

PER SERVING

½ [✴] Sugar Choice
½ [▲] Fat & Oil Choice

Calories 36
Carbohydrates . . . . . 3 g
Fiber . . . . 0 g
Protein . . . . 0 g
Fat, total . . . . 3 g
Fat, saturated . . . . 0 g
Sodium . . . . 1 mg
Cholesterol . . . . . . 0 mg

Makes 1⅓ cups
(325 mL)

Toss with pasta or
serve over cooked fish
or chicken.

◆

If sauce is too thick, add
a little water to thin.

◆

This sauce makes
enough for 1½ lb
(750 g) pasta.

◆

This sauce is a good
source of vitamin C.
Tomatoes are also a
good source of lycopene,
the red pigment which
gives tomato products
their color. Lycopene is a
phytochemical which
some research indicates
may be associated with
reduced risk of some
kinds of cancers.

Sun-Dried Tomato Sauce

4 oz	sun-dried tomatoes	125 g
1 tsp	crushed garlic	5 mL
¾ cup	water or chicken stock	175 mL
½ cup	chopped fresh parsley	125 mL
2 tbsp	olive oil	25 mL
2 tbsp	toasted pine nuts	25 mL
1 tbsp	grated Parmesan cheese	15 mL

1. In bowl, pour enough boiling water over tomatoes to cover; let sit for 15 minutes or until soft enough to cut. Cut into smaller pieces.

2. In food processor, combine tomatoes, garlic, water, parsley, oil, pine nuts and cheese; process until well blended.

PER SERVING

| ☑ Fruit & Vegetable Choice |
| ▲ Fat & Oil Choice |

Calories 73
Carbohydrates . . . . . 8 g
Fiber . . . . 0 g
Protein . . . . 3 g
Fat, total . . . . 4 g
Fat, saturated . . . . 1 g
Sodium . . . . 314 mg
Cholesterol . . . . . . 1 mg

Pesto Sauce

½ cup	well-packed chopped fresh parsley	125 mL
½ cup	well-packed chopped fresh basil	125 mL
¼ cup	water or chicken stock	50 mL
1 tbsp	toasted pine nuts	15 mL
2 tbsp	grated Parmesan cheese	25 mL
3 tbsp	olive oil	45 mL
¾ tsp	crushed garlic	4 mL

1. In food processor, combine parsley, basil, water, pine nuts, Parmesan, oil and garlic; process until smooth.

MAKE AHEAD ◆ Refrigerate for up to a week or freeze for up to 6 weeks.

PER SERVING

½ ▲ Fat & Oil Choice

Calories	37
Carbohydrates	0 g
Fiber	0 g
Protein	1 g
Fat, total	4 g
Fat, saturated	1 g
Sodium	21 mg
Cholesterol	1 mg

If they're available, use wild mushrooms, such as chanterelle or oyster.

◆

Serve over cooked beef, chicken or pork.

◆

This flavorful mushroom sauce has much less fat than others which might be commercially available.

Mushroom Sauce

1 tbsp	margarine	15 mL
1½ cups	sliced mushrooms	375 mL
2 tbsp	all-purpose flour	25 mL
½ cup	chicken or beef stock	125 mL
½ cup	2% milk	125 mL
1 tbsp	sherry (optional)	5 mL

1. In small nonstick saucepan, melt margarine; sauté mushrooms until tender, approximately 3 minutes. Add flour and stir until combined.

2. Add stock and milk; cook on low heat, stirring constantly, until thickened, 4 to 5 minutes. Add sherry (if using). If too thick add more milk.

MAKE AHEAD ◆ Prepare and refrigerate up to a day before, then gently reheat.

PER SERVING

½ ◢ Fruit & Vegetable Choice

½ ▲ Fat & Oil Choice

Calories	32
Carbohydrates	3 g
Fiber	0 g
Protein	1 g
Fat, total	2 g
Fat, saturated	0 g
Sodium	112 mg
Cholesterol	1 mg

Desserts

The Canadian Diabetes Association nutrition guidelines for diabetes suggest that up to 10% of the total calories in the diet can come from "added sugars". The recipes contained in this section use regular sugar instead of sugar substitutes.

Using sugar substitutes can maintain the sweetness, but may alter the texture in baked goods.

If you wish to reduce the sugar or carbohydrate content of these recipes, begin by choosing recipes such as Mango Blueberry Strudel (page 173) or the Individual Miniature Cheesecakes (page 180). One quarter cup of sugar contains 50 g of carbohydrate or equals five ✳ Sugars Choices. Keep this in mind when making alterations to the Food Choice Values or carbohydrate content of the recipe.

❖

Makes 20 half slices

Preheat oven to 350°F (180°C)

9- x 5- inch (2 L) loaf pan sprayed with nonstick vegetable spray

TIPS

You can also make muffins by pouring batter into 12 cups and baking in 375°F (190°C) oven for 15 to 20 minutes.

◆

If you like a strong lemon taste, use 1 tsp (5 mL) more lemon rind.

◆

In this recipe, granulated sugar is used in the loaf and icing sugar is used in the glaze. When using this loaf, 1 ☀ Sugar Choice can replace 1 ✐ Fruit & Vegetable Choice in your meal plan.

PER SERVING

½ ◼ Starch Choice
1 ☀ Sugar Choice
½ ▲ Fat & Oil Choice

Calories 102
Carbohydrates . . . . 16 g
Fiber . . . . 1 g
Protein . . . . 2 g
Fat, total . . . . 4 g
Fat, saturated . . . . 1 g
Sodium . . . . 88 mg
Cholesterol . . . . . 11 mg

Lemon Poppy Seed Loaf

¾ cup	granulated sugar	175 mL
⅓ cup	soft margarine	75 mL
1	egg	1
2 tsp	grated lemon rind	10 mL
3 tbsp	lemon juice	45 mL
⅓ cup	2% milk	75 mL
1¼ cups	all-purpose flour	300 mL
1 tbsp	poppy seeds	15 mL
1 tsp	baking powder	5 mL
½ tsp	baking soda	2 mL
⅓ cup	2% yogurt or light sour cream	75 mL

GLAZE

¼ cup	icing sugar	50 mL
2 tbsp	lemon juice	25 mL

1. In large bowl or food processor, beat together sugar, margarine, egg, lemon rind and juice, mixing well. Add milk, mixing well.

2. Combine flour, poppy seeds, baking powder and baking soda; add to bowl alternately with yogurt, mixing just until incorporated. Do not overmix. Pour into pan and bake for 35 to 40 minutes or until tester inserted into center comes out dry.

3. Glaze: Prick holes in top of loaf with fork. Combine icing sugar with lemon juice; pour over loaf.

MAKE AHEAD ◆ Bake a day before or freeze for up to 6 weeks.

Makes 20 slices

Preheat oven to 375°F (190°C)

9- x 5-inch (2 L) loaf pan sprayed with nonstick vegetable spray

TIP

If you like muffins, fill 12 muffin cups and bake approximately 20 minutes or until tops are firm to the touch.

Banana Nut Raisin Loaf

2	large ripe bananas	2
⅓ cup	soft margarine	75 mL
½ cup	granulated sugar	125 mL
1	egg	1
1	egg white	1
¼ cup	hot water	50 mL
1⅓ cups	whole wheat flour	325 mL
¾ tsp	baking soda	4 mL
¼ cup	raisins	50 mL
⅓ cup	chopped pecans or walnuts	75 mL

1. In bowl or food processor, beat bananas and margarine; beat in sugar, egg, egg white and water until smooth.

2. Combine flour and baking soda; stir into batter along with raisins and all but a few of the pecans, mixing just until blended. Do not overmix. Pour into pan; arrange reserved nuts down middle of mixture. Bake for 35 to 45 minutes or until tester inserted into center comes out dry.

MAKE AHEAD ◆ Make up to 2 days in advance or freeze for up to 2 months.

PER SERVING

½ ▪ Starch Choice

½ ◗ Fruit & Vegetable Choice

1 ▲ Fat & Oil Choice

Calories 107
Carbohydrates . . . . 16 g
Fiber . . . . 1 g
Protein . . . . 2 g
Fat, total . . . . 5 g
Fat, saturated . . . . 1 g
Sodium . . . . 84 mg
Cholesterol . . . . . 11 mg

Makes 20 slices

Preheat oven to 350°F (180°C)

9- x 5-inch (2 L) loaf pan sprayed with nonstick vegetable spray

PER SERVING

½	▣	Starch Choice
½	◪	Fruit & Vegetable Choice
1	✳	Sugar Choice
½	▲	Fat & Oil Choice

Calories	119
Carbohydrates	22 g
Fiber	3 g
Protein	2 g
Fat, total	3 g
Fat, saturated	0 g
Sodium	116 mg
Cholesterol	11 mg

Carrot Pineapple Zucchini Loaf

¼ cup	margarine	50 mL
1 cup	granulated sugar	250 mL
1	egg	1
1	egg white	1
2 tsp	cinnamon	10 mL
1½ tsp	vanilla	7 mL
¼ tsp	nutmeg	1 mL
¾ cup	grated carrot	175 mL
¾ cup	grated zucchini	175 mL
½ cup	drained crushed pineapple	125 mL
⅓ cup	raisins	75 mL
1¼ cups	all-purpose flour	300 mL
½ cup	whole wheat flour	125 mL
1 tsp	baking powder	5 mL
1 tsp	baking soda	5 mL

1. In large bowl or food processor, cream margarine with sugar. Add egg, egg white, cinnamon, vanilla and nutmeg; beat well. Stir in carrot, zucchini, pineapple and raisins, blending until well combined.

2. Combine all-purpose and whole wheat flours, baking powder and soda; add to bowl and mix just until combined. Pour into loaf pan and bake for 35 to 45 minutes or until tester inserted into center comes out dry.

MAKE AHEAD ◆ Make up to 2 days in advance or freeze for up to 2 months.

Preheat oven to 350°F (180°C)

9- by 5-inch (2 L) loaf pan sprayed with vegetable spray

TIPS

Grate carrots or chop and process them in food processor just until finely diced. Chopped, pitted dates can replace raisins.

◆

Orange fruits and vegetables such carrots, squash, mangoes are good sources of beta carotene or vitamin A.

PER SERVING

½ ■ Starch Choice

½ ◢ Fruit & Vegetable Choice

½ ✴ Sugar Choice

1 ▲ Fat & Oil Choice

Calories 111
Carbohydrates . . . . 17 g
Fiber . . . . 1 g
Protein . . . . 2 g
Fat, total. . . . . 4 g
Fat, saturated . . . . 2 g
Sodium . . . . 121 mg
Cholesterol . . . . . 22 mg

Carrot, Apple and Coconut Loaf

⅔ cup	granulated sugar	150 mL
¼ cup	margarine or butter	50 mL
2	eggs	2
1½ tsp	cinnamon	7 mL
¼ tsp	nutmeg	1 mL
1 tsp	vanilla	5 mL
1¼ cup	grated carrots	300 mL
⅔ cup	peeled, finely chopped apples	150 mL
⅓ cup	unsweetened shredded coconut	75 mL
⅓ cup	raisins	75 mL
⅔ cup	all-purpose flour	150 mL
½ cup	whole wheat flour	125 mL
1 tsp	baking powder	5 mL
1 tsp	baking soda	5 mL
⅓ cup	2% yogurt	75 mL

1. In large bowl or food processor, cream together sugar and margarine. Add eggs, cinnamon, nutmeg and vanilla; beat well. Stir in carrots, apples, coconut and raisins.

2. In bowl, combine flour, whole wheat flour, baking powder and baking soda; add to batter alternately with yogurt, mixing until just combined. Pour batter into loaf pan; bake for 40 to 45 minutes or until tester inserted in center comes out clean.

MAKE AHEAD ◆ Prepare up to a day ahead, or freeze up to 4 weeks.

Preheat oven to 375°F
(190°C)
12 muffin cups
sprayed with nonstick
vegetable spray

Streusel Apple and Raisin Muffins

½ cup	brown sugar	125 mL
½ cup	applesauce	125 mL
¼ cup	vegetable oil	50 mL
1	egg	1
1 tsp	vanilla	5 mL
1 cup	all-purpose flour	250 mL
1 tsp	baking soda	5 mL
1 tsp	baking powder	5 mL
½ tsp	cinnamon	2 mL
¾ cup	diced peeled apple	175 mL

TOPPING

2 tbsp	brown sugar	25 mL
2 tsp	all-purpose flour	10 mL
½ tsp	cinnamon	2 mL
1 tsp	margarine	5 mL

1. In large bowl, combine sugar, applesauce, oil, egg and vanilla until well mixed. Combine flour, baking soda, baking powder and cinnamon; stir into bowl just until incorporated. Stir in apple. Pour into muffin cups, filling two-thirds full.

2. Topping: In small bowl, combine sugar, flour and cinnamon; cut in margarine until crumbly. Sprinkle evenly over muffins. Bake for 20 minutes or until tops are firm to the touch.

MAKE AHEAD ◆ Prepare up to a day before. Freeze for up to 6 weeks.

PER SERVING

½	■	Starch Choice
½	◪	Fruit & Vegetable Choice
1	✽	Sugar Choice
1	▲	Fat & Oil Choice

Calories 156
Carbohydrates . . . . 26 g
Fiber . . . . 1 g
Protein . . . . 2 g
Fat, total . . . . 6 g
Fat, saturated . . . . 1 g
Sodium . . . . 144 mg
Cholesterol . . . . . 18 mg

Preheat oven to 375°F (190°C)

12 muffin cups sprayed with nonstick vegetable spray

A 9- x 5-inch (2 L) loaf pan can also be used; bake for 30 to 40 minutes or until tester comes out dry.

◆

Use the ripest bananas possible for the best flavor.

Blueberry Banana Muffins

¾ cup	puréed bananas (about 1 ½ bananas)	175 mL
½ cup	granulated sugar	125 mL
⅓ cup	vegetable oil	75 mL
1	egg	1
1 tsp	vanilla	5 mL
1 cup	all-purpose flour	250 mL
1 tsp	baking powder	5 mL
1 tsp	baking soda	5 mL
¼ cup	2% yogurt or light sour cream	50 mL
½ cup	blueberries	125 mL

1. In large bowl, beat together bananas, sugar, oil, egg and vanilla until well mixed.

2. Combine flour, baking powder and baking soda; stir into bowl. Stir in yogurt; fold in blueberries.

3. Pour batter into muffin cups; bake for approximately 20 minutes or until tops are firm to the touch.

MAKE AHEAD ◆ Bake a day before or freeze for up to 6 weeks.

PER SERVING

½ ▣ Starch Choice

½ ◪ Fruit & Vegetable Choice

1 ✳ Sugar Choice

1 ½ ▲ Fat & Oil Choices

Calories 151
Carbohydrates . . . . 21 g
Fiber . . . . 1 g
Protein . . . . 2 g
Fat, total . . . . 7 g
Fat, saturated . . . . . . 1 g
Sodium . . . . 138 mg
Cholesterol . . . . . 18 mg

Preheat oven to 350°F (180°C)

Baking sheet sprayed with nonstick vegetable spray

TIPS

This decadent strudel is a wonderful finish to a dinner with guests.

◆

Ripen pears at room temperature in a bowl or paper bag.

Pear, Apple and Raisin Strudel

2²/₃ cups	chopped peeled apples	650 mL
2²/₃ cups	chopped peeled pears	650 mL
¹/₃ cup	raisins	75 mL
2 tbsp	chopped pecans or walnuts	25 mL
2 tbsp	brown sugar	25 mL
1 tbsp	lemon juice	15 mL
1 tbsp	honey	15 mL
1 tsp	cinnamon	5 mL
6	phyllo sheets	6
4 tsp	margarine, melted	20 mL

1. In bowl, combine apples, pears, raisins, pecans, sugar, lemon juice, honey and cinnamon; mix well.

2. Lay out 2 sheets of phyllo; brush with some margarine. Place 2 more sheets over top; brush with margarine again. Top with remaining 2 sheets phyllo.

3. Spread filling over phyllo, leaving 1-inch (2.5 cm) border uncovered. Roll up like jelly roll and place seam down on baking sheet. Brush with remaining margarine. Bake for 40 to 50 minutes or until golden and fruit is tender.

MAKE AHEAD ◆ Filling can be prepared a couple of hours before baking. Keep covered. Do not assemble strudel until ready to bake.

PER SERVING

½ ■ Starch Choice

1½ ▨ Fruit & Vegetable Choices

½ ✳ Sugar Choice

½ ▲ Fat & Oil Choice

Calories 142
Carbohydrates . . . . 29 g
Fiber . . . . 3 g
Protein . . . . 1 g
Fat, total . . . . 3 g
Fat, saturated . . . . 0 g
Sodium . . . . 75 mg
Cholesterol . . . . . . 0 mg

Preheat oven to 375°F (190°C)

Baking sheet sprayed with vegetable spray

TIPS

Mango can be replaced with ripe peaches or even pears.

◆

Phyllo pastry is located in the freezer section of store. Handle quickly so the sheets do not dry out. Cover those not being used with a slightly damp cloth.

Mango Blueberry Strudel

2 cups	fresh blueberries (or frozen, thawed and drained)	500 mL
1 tbsp	all-purpose flour	15 mL
2½ cups	peeled chopped ripe mango	625 mL
¼ cup	granulated sugar	50 mL
1 tbsp	lemon juice	15 mL
½ tsp	cinnamon	2 mL
6	sheets phyllo pastry	6
2 tsp	melted margarine or butter	10 mL

1. Toss blueberries with flour. In large bowl, combine mango, blueberries, sugar, lemon juice and cinnamon.

2. Lay 2 phyllo sheets one on top of the other; brush with melted margarine. Layer another 2 phyllo sheets on top and brush with melted margarine. Layer last 2 sheets on top. Put fruit filling along long end of phyllo; gently roll over until all of filling is enclosed, fold sides in, and continue to roll. Put on prepared baking sheet, brush with remaining margarine and bake for 20 to 25 minutes or until golden. Sprinkle with icing sugar.

MAKE AHEAD ◆ Prepare filling early in the day. For best results, do not fill until just ready to bake. If in a hurry, fill phyllo, cover and refrigerate. Bake just ahead serving.

PER SERVING

½ ■ Starch Choice

1½ ◪ Fruit & Vegetable Choices

½ ✳ Sugar Choice

½ ▲ Fat & Oil Choice

Calories 147
Carbohydrates . . . . 31 g
Fiber . . . . 2 g
Protein . . . . 2 g
Fat, total . . . . 2 g
Fat, saturated . . . . 0 g
Sodium . . . . 101 mg
Cholesterol . . . . . . 0 mg

Makes 40 cookies

Preheat oven to 350°F (180°C)

Baking sheets sprayed with nonstick vegetable spray

Peanut Butter Chocolate Chip Cookies

½ cup	brown sugar	125 mL
⅓ cup	granulated sugar	75 mL
⅓ cup	peanut butter	75 mL
⅓ cup	2% milk	75 mL
¼ cup	soft margarine	50 mL
I	egg	I
I tsp	vanilla	5 mL
½ cup	all-purpose flour	125 mL
⅓ cup	whole wheat flour	75 mL
I tsp	baking soda	5 mL
⅓ cup	chocolate chips	75 mL
¼ cup	raisins	50 mL

I. In large bowl or food processor, beat together brown and granulated sugars, peanut butter, milk, margarine, egg and vanilla until well blended.

2. Combine all-purpose and whole wheat flours and baking soda; add to bowl and mix just until incorporated. Do not overmix. Stir in chocolate chips and raisins.

3. Drop by heaping teaspoonfuls (5 mL) 2 inches (5 cm) apart onto baking sheets. Bake for 12 to 15 minutes or until browned.

MAKE AHEAD ◆ Dough can be frozen up to 2 weeks. Bake just before eating for best flavor.

PER SERVING	
I	✱ Sugar Choice
½	▲ Fat & Oil Choice

Calories	70
Carbohydrates	10 g
Fiber	I g
Protein	I g
Fat, total	3 g
Fat, saturated	I g
Sodium	51 mg
Cholesterol	6 mg

Makes 30 cookies

Preheat oven to 350°F (180°C)

Baking sheets sprayed with nonstick vegetable spray

Oatmeal Raisin Pecan Cookies

½ cup	brown sugar	125 mL
¼ cup	soft margarine	50 mL
1	egg	1
1 tsp	vanilla	5 mL
½ cup	rolled oats	125 mL
¼ cup	whole wheat flour	50 mL
¼ cup	wheat germ	50 mL
¼ cup	pecan pieces	50 mL
¼ cup	raisins	50 mL
½ tsp	baking powder	2 mL

1. In large bowl or food processor, beat together sugar, margarine, egg and vanilla until well blended.

2. Add rolled oats, flour, wheat germ, pecans, raisins and baking powder; mix just until incorporated.

3. Drop by heaping teaspoonfuls (5 mL) 2 inches (5 cm) apart onto baking sheets. Bake for 12 to 15 minutes or until browned.

MAKE AHEAD ♦ Dough can be frozen for up to 2 weeks.

PER SERVING

½ ■ Starch Choice

½ ▲ Fat & Oil Choice

Calories	57
Carbohydrates	8 g
Fiber	0 g
Protein	1 g
Fat, total	3 g
Fat, saturated	0 g
Sodium	27 mg
Cholesterol	7 mg

Preheat oven to 350°F
(180°C)

Baking sheet sprayed
with nonstick
vegetable spray

TIP

This cookie dough can
be chilled, then rolled
out and cut into
various patterns.

Cinnamon Ginger Cookies

¼ cup	brown sugar	50 mL
3 tbsp	margarine, melted	45 mL
2 tbsp	molasses	25 mL
2 tbsp	2% yogurt	25 mL
1 tsp	vanilla	5 mL
1 cup	all-purpose flour	250 mL
½ tsp	baking soda	2 mL
½ tsp	ginger	2 mL
½ tsp	cinnamon	2 mL
Pinch	nutmeg	Pinch
1½ tsp	brown sugar	7 mL

1. In bowl, combine ¼ cup (50 mL) brown sugar, margarine, molasses, yogurt and vanilla until well mixed.

2. Combine flour, baking soda, ginger, cinnamon and nutmeg; stir into bowl just until combined.

3. Using teaspoon, form dough into small balls and place on baking sheet. Press flat with fork; sprinkle with 1½ tsp (7 mL) brown sugar. Bake for 10 to 12 minutes.

MAKE AHEAD ◆ Dough can be frozen for up to 2 weeks.

**PER SERVING
(2 COOKIES)**

½ ■ Starch Choice

½ ✳ Sugar Choice

½ ▲ Fat & Oil Choice

Calories 76
Carbohydrates . . . . 12 g
Fiber . . . . 0 g
Protein . . . . 1 g
Fat, total . . . . 2 g
Fat, saturated . . . . 0 g
Sodium . . . . 68 mg
Cholesterol . . . . . . 0 mg

Makes about 32 cookies

Preheat oven to 350°F
(180°C)

Large baking sheet
sprayed with
vegetable spray

TIPS

For maximum freshness,
store cookies in airtight
containers in the freezer;
remove as needed.

◆

Try this recipe with dried
figs or apricots.

◆

In this recipe, the dates
contribute more
carbohydrate than the
added sugar. Two dates
are 1 ■ Fruit &
Vegetable choice or
provide 10 g of
carbohydrate. Keeping
blood sugars down
means thinking about
both added sugars as
well as those from
other sources.

PER SERVING

½ ■ Starch Choice
½ ◢ Fruit & Vegetable
Choice
1 ▲ Fat & Oil Choice

Calories 106
Carbohydrates . . . . 17 g
Fiber . . . . 1 g
Protein . . . . 1 g
Fat, total . . . . 4 g
Fat, saturated . . . . 0 g
Sodium . . . . 20 mg
Cholesterol . . . . . . 0 mg

Date Roll-Up Cookies

FILLING

8 oz	pitted dried dates	250 g
1 cup	orange juice	250 mL
¼ tsp	ground cinnamon	1 mL

DOUGH

2¼ cups	all-purpose flour	550 mL
⅔ cup	granulated sugar	150 mL
¼ cup	margarine or butter	50 mL
¼ cup	vegetable oil	50 mL
¼ cup	2% plain yogurt	50 mL
3 tbsp	water	45 mL
1 tsp	vanilla extract	5 mL
1 tsp	grated orange zest	5 mL

1. Make the filling: In a saucepan bring dates,
orange juice and cinnamon to a boil; reduce heat
to medium-low and cook 10 minutes or until soft.
Mash with a fork until liquid is absorbed. Refrigerate.

2. Make the dough: In a food processor, combine
flour, sugar, margarine, oil, yogurt, water, vanilla
and orange zest; process until dough forms. Add up
to 1 tbsp (15 mL) more water, if necessary. Divide
dough in half; form each half into a ball, wrap and
refrigerate for 15 minutes or until chilled.

3. Between 2 sheets of waxed paper sprinkled with
flour, roll one of the dough balls into a rectangle,
approximately 12 by 10 inches (30 by 25 cm) and ⅛
inch (5 mm) thick. Remove top sheet of waxed
paper. Spread half of date mixture over rolled
dough. Starting at short end and using the waxed
paper as an aid, roll up tightly. Cut into ½-inch
(1 cm) slices and place on prepared baking sheet.
Repeat with remaining dough and filling.

4. Bake 25 minutes or until lightly browned.

MAKE AHEAD ◆ Prepare date mixture and freeze
until needed.

Preheat oven to 350°F
(180°C)

Baking sheet sprayed
with vegetable spray

Two-Tone Chocolate Orange Biscotti

1¼ cups	granulated sugar	300 mL
⅓ cup	margarine or butter	75 mL
2	eggs	2
2 tbsp	orange juice concentrate	25 mL
1 tbsp	grated orange zest	15 mL
2⅔ cups	all-purpose flour	650 mL
2½ tsp	baking powder	12 mL
3 tbsp	cocoa	45 mL

1. In a food processor or in a bowl with an electric mixer, beat together sugar, margarine, eggs, orange juice concentrate and orange zest until smooth. Add flour and baking powder; mix just until combined.

2. Divide dough in half; to one half, add cocoa and mix well. Divide chocolate and plain doughs in half to produce 4 doughs. Roll each piece into a long thin rope approximately 12 inches (30 cm) long and 1 inch (2.5 cm) wide. Use extra flour if too sticky. Place 1 cocoa dough on top of (or beside) each plain dough. (Ensure the plain and cocoa doughs touch one another.)

3. Bake 20 minutes. Cool 10 minutes. Cut logs on an angle into ½-inch (1 cm) slices. Bake another 20 minutes.

MAKE AHEAD ◆ Freeze in containers for up to 6 weeks.

PER SERVING

1   ✱ Sugar Choice

½   ▲ Fat & Oil Choice

Calories	61
Carbohydrates	11 g
Fiber	0 g
Protein	1 g
Fat, total	2 g
Fat, saturated	0 g
Sodium	32 mg
Cholesterol	9 mg

9-inch (2.5 L) square
baking dish sprayed
with vegetable spray

Sift some cocoa on top
of each portion just
before serving. This
tiramisu tastes so
decadent, you'll never
believe it hasn't the
same calories and fat
as the one made
with mascarpone.

◆

Spongy or harder lady
fingers can be used.

◆

The longer this chills,
the better it is. The
liqueur-coffee mixture
penetrates the cookies.

Chocolate Coffee Tiramisu

1½ cups	5% ricotta cheese	375 mL
½ cup	light cream cheese	125 mL
½ cup	granulated sugar	125 mL
3 tbsp	cocoa	45 mL
1	egg yolk	1
1 tsp	vanilla	5 mL
3	egg whites	3
⅓ cup	granulated sugar	75 mL
¾ cup	strong, prepared coffee	175 mL
3 tbsp	chocolate or coffee-flavored liqueur	45 mL
16	lady finger cookies	16

1. In food processor, combine ricotta cheese, cream cheese, sugar, cocoa, egg yolk and vanilla until smooth; transfer to a bowl.

2. In bowl, beat egg whites until soft peaks form. Gradually add sugar and continue to beat until stiff peaks form. Gently fold the whites into the ricotta mixture.

3. Combine coffee and liqueur in a small bowl.

4. Put half of lady fingers in bottom of dish. Sprinkle with half of coffee-liqueur mixture. Spread half of ricotta mixture on top. Repeat layers. Cover and chill for at least 3 hours, or overnight.

MAKE AHEAD ◆ Prepare up to 2 days ahead. It tastes best after 8 hours of refrigeration.

PER SERVING

½ ▣ Starch Choice

1½ ❋ Sugar Choices

½ ◲ Protein Choice

½ ▲ Fat & Oil Choice

Calories 150
Carbohydrates . . . . 21 g
Fiber . . . . 0 g
Protein . . . . 6 g
Fat, total . . . . 5 g
Fat, saturated . . . . 2 g
Sodium . . . . 102 mg
Cholesterol . . . . . 66 mg

Preheat oven to 350°F
(180°C)

Line 10 muffin cups
with muffin paper cups

TIPS

Substitute one 8-oz
(250 g) package of light
cream cheese for the
ricotta cheese.

◆

Decorate cheesecakes
with berries and sliced
fresh fruit; glaze with
2 tbsp (25 mL) no sugar
added apricot spread.

◆

Count fruit topping
as a ◢ Fruit &
Vegetable Choice.

Individual Miniature Cheesecakes

1 cup	5% ricotta cheese	250 mL
1 cup	low-fat cottage cheese	250 mL
⅓ cup	granulated sugar	75 mL
1	medium egg	1
¼ cup	light sour cream	50 mL
½ tsp	cornstarch	2 mL
⅛ tsp	vanilla extract	0.5 mL
	Fruit purée (optional)	

1. In a food processor, combine ricotta cheese, cottage cheese and sugar; purée until smooth. Beat in egg. Blend in sour cream, cornstarch and vanilla until well mixed. Divide batter among muffin cups. Set muffin tin in larger pan; pour in enough hot water to come half way up sides. Bake 30 to 35 minutes or until tester inserted in center comes out clean. Remove from water bath; cool on wire rack. Chill.

2. Serve with fruit purée, if desired.

PER SERVING

1	✳ Sugar Choice
1	◢ Protein Choice
1	▲ Fat & Oil Choice

Calories 127
Carbohydrates . . . . . 9 g
Fiber . . . . 0 g
Protein . . . . 6 g
Fat, total . . . . 8 g
Fat, saturated . . . . 4 g
Sodium . . . . 268 mg
Cholesterol . . . . . 42 mg

Add 1 tsp (5 mL) each lemon extract and grated lemon rind to make lemon yogurt.

Frozen Vanilla Yogurt

1	egg	1
⅓ cup	brown sugar	75 mL
½ cup	2% milk	125 mL
1 ½ cups	2% yogurt	375 mL
1 ½ tsp	vanilla	7 mL

1. In bowl, beat egg with sugar until combined; set aside. In saucepan, heat milk just until bubbles appear around side of pan. Stir a little into egg mixture, then pour back into saucepan. Cook over low heat, stirring, just until thickened, 2 to 4 minutes. (Do not let boil or egg will curdle.) Remove from heat and let cool completely.

2. Beat yogurt and vanilla into cooled mixture. Freeze in ice-cream machine according to manufacturer's directions. (Or pour into cake pan and freeze until nearly solid. Chop into chunks and beat with electric mixer or process in food processor until smooth. Freeze again until solid.)

MAKE AHEAD ◆ This dessert can be prepared up to 2 days in advance, but it is best if served right after freezing.

PER SERVING

1	◆ 2% Milk Choice
1	✳ Sugar Choice

Calories 114
Carbohydrates . . . . 17 g
Fiber . . . . 0 g
Protein . . . . 5 g
Fat, total . . . . 3 g
Fat, saturated . . . . . . 2 g
Sodium . . . . 60 mg
Cholesterol . . . . . 43 mg

This is a delicious tropical low-fat finish to a meal.

◆

If you don't have an ice cream maker, pour into a baking dish and freeze until solid. Break into small pieces; in a food processor, pulse on and off until smooth. Store in freezer until ready to serve.

◆

Purée canned crushed pineapple for the smoothest texture.

Pineapple Lime Sorbet

1 ¼ cups	pineapple purée	300 mL
2 tsp	grated lime or lemon zest	10 mL
¾ cup	freshly squeezed lime or lemon juice	175 mL
¼ cup	water	50 mL
	Thin slices lime or lemon	

1. In a bowl, stir together pineapple purée, lime zest and juice, water and, if desired, sugar.

2. In an ice cream maker, freeze according to manufacturer's directions.

3. Divide among 4 individual dessert dishes. Serve garnished with thin slices of lime.

PER SERVING

1	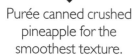 Fruit & Vegetable Choice
Calories............38	
Carbohydrates ....11 g	
Fiber...............1 g	
Protein............1 g	
Fat, total...........0 g	
Fat, saturated.......0 g	
Sodium...........1 mg	
Cholesterol......0 mg	

Use fresh ripe strawberries or unsweetened frozen berries; if using frozen, thaw and drain before using.

◆

For attractive orange segments, peel a whole orange with a sharp knife, removing zest, pith and membrane; cut on both sides of dividing membranes to release segments.

◆

This mousse is an excellent source of vitamin C, providing half of the daily recommended amount.

Banana-Strawberry Mousse

3	small ripe bananas	3
1 cup	orange juice	250 mL
1 cup	strawberries	250 mL
6 tbsp	lemon juice	90 mL
½ cup	cold water	125 mL
1	pkg (1 tbsp [7 g]) gelatin	1
	Orange segments or sliced strawberries	

1. In a blender, combine bananas, orange juice, strawberries and lemon juice; purée until smooth. Put water in a small saucepan; sprinkle with gelatin. Let stand 1 minute. Heat gently, stirring until gelatin dissolves. With motor running, pour hot gelatin through blender feed tube; purée until smooth. Divide among 6 individual dessert dishes or champagne coupes.

2. Chill 2 hours. Serve garnished with orange segments or sliced strawberries.

PER SERVING

2 ◢ Fruit & Vegetable Choices

Calories 88
Carbohydrates . . . . 21 g
Fiber . . . . 2 g
Protein . . . . 2 g
Fat, total . . . . 0.4 g
Fat, saturated . . . . 0 g
Sodium . . . . 4 mg
Cholesterol . . . . . . 0 mg

National Library of Canada Cataloguing in Publication Data

Main entry under title:
The diabetes choice cookbook for Canadians

Includes index.
ISBN 0-7788-0043-1

1. Diabetes—Diet therapy—Recipes.
I. Younker, Katherine E.

RC662.D5195 2002   641.5'6314   C2001-903479-2

Index

Orange
  balsamic vinaigrette,
    158
  chocolate biscotti, 178
  dressing, 66–67, 69
Orange roughy, pasta
    pizza with goat
    cheese, 84–85
Oriental-style
  beef bundles in lettuce,
    105
  chicken wrapped
    mushrooms, 29
  vegetable salad, 61
Orzo, Greek-style seafood
    salad, 64

P
Parmesan cheese
  asparagus and leek soup,
    47
  broccoli and lentil soup,
    50
  Caesar dressing, 63
  Caesar pasta salad, 127
  cherry tomatoes stuffed
    with, 30
  chicken and eggplant
    with, 95
  chicken livers with
    rigatoni, 99
  cream sauce, 90–91
  creamy sun-dried tomato
    dip, 37
  dill artichoke bake, 36
  halibut with lemon and
    pecans, 75
  macaroni and cheese,
    108
  meatballs, 111
  pasta shells filled with
    smoked salmon and,
    123
  pasta with squid and
    clams in tomato sauce,
    86
  pesto
    dip, 38
    potato salad, 70–71
    sauce, 163

roasted garlic sweet
    peppers, 147
  rotini with tomatoes
    and, 121
  scallops with basil
    tomato sauce, 83
  seafood pasta pizza
    with goat cheese,
    84–85
  spinach quiche, 154
  stuffed baked potatoes,
    152
  sun-dried tomato sauce,
    97
  tuna and white bean
    spread, 40
  white fish crunchy fillets,
    80
Parsley, pesto sauce,
    163
Pasta
  chili, chicken and pasta
    stew, 55
  and clam chowder, 54
  pizza, seafood with goat
    cheese, 84–85
  salad with apricots and
    dates, 69
  with squid and clams in
    tomato sauce, 86
  stew with meatballs,
    124–25
  sun-dried tomato and
    leek bake, 126
  with turkey tomato
    sauce, 119
  See also specific varieties
    of pasta
Pâté, leek mushroom
    cheese, 39
Peanut butter, chocolate
    chip cookies, 174
Pear
  apple and raisin strudel,
    172
  lettuce and feta cheese
    salad, 58
Pearl barley. See Barley
Pecans, to toast, 65, 75,
    145

Penne
  with Brie cheese and
    tomatoes, 67
  Caesar salad, 127
  chicken Tetrazzini, 100
  vegetables over, 150
  with wild mushrooms,
    149
Pesto
  lamb stuffed with rice
    and, 115
  potato salad, 70–71
  salmon with, 74
  sauce, 118, 163
  stuffed mushrooms, 151
Phyllo pastry
  strudel, 172, 173
  tip, 173
Pine nuts
  linguine with shrimp
    and red peppers, 87
  pesto potato salad, 70–71
  pesto sauce, 163
  to toast, 37, 38, 118, 151
Pineapple lime
  sauce, 112
  sorbet, 182
Pizza pasta
  with beef-tomato sauce,
    109
  seafood with goat
    cheese, 84–85
Polenta, with chèvre and
    roasted vegetables, 134
Polynesian wild rice salad,
    66–67
Poppy seed dressing, 159
Pork
  ground
    chili bean and pasta
      stew, 55
    ratatouille chili, 102
  loin, stir-fry, 113
  with mango salsa, 79
  scallopini
    and eggplant Parmesan,
      95
    with pineapple lime
      sauce, 112
  tenderloin, fajitas, 114